27 Update in Intensive Care and Emergency Medicine

Edited by J.-L. Vincent

Springer
Berlin
Heidelberg
New York
Barcelona
Budapest
Hong Kong
London
Milan
Paris
Santa Clara
Singapore
Tokyo

T. Steiner W. Hacke D. F. Hanley (Eds.)

Stroke

Emergency Management and Critical Care

With 108 Figures and 15 Tables

Springer

Series Editor

Prof. Dr. Jean-Louis Vincent
Clinical Director, Department of Intensive Care
Erasme University Hospital
Route de Lennik 808, B-1070 Brussels, Belgium

Volume Editors

Dr. Thorsten Steiner
Prof. Dr. Werner Hacke
Universität Heidelberg, Neurologische Klinik
Im Neuenheimer Feld 400, D-69120 Heidelberg, Germany

Prof. Dr. Daniel F. Hanley
John Hopkins University, Medical School
Division of Neurosciences Critical Care
600 North Wolfe Str/Meyer 8-140, 21287-7840 Baltimore, MD, USA

ISSN 0933-6788

ISBN-13: 978-3-642-64326-2 Springer-Verlag Berlin Heidelberg New York

Library of Congress Cataloging-in-Publication Data
Stroke : emergency management and critical care / Th. Steiner, W. Hacke, D. F. Hanley (eds.). (Update in intensive care and emergency medicine ; 27) Includes bibliographical references and index. ISBN-13: 978-3-642-64326-2(softcover: alk. paper) 1. Cerebrovascular disease. 2. Medical emergencies. 3. Critical care medicine. I. Steiner, Thorsten, 1961- . II. Hanley, D. F. (Daniel F.), 1949- . III. Hacke, W. (Werner), 1948- . IV. Series. [DNLM: 1. Cerebrovascular Disorders--therapy. 2. Critical Care--methods. 3. Emergency Medical Services--methods. W1 UP66H v.27 1998 / WL 355 S91913 1998] RC388.5.S85238 1998 616.89--dc21 DNLM/DLC

ISBN-13: 978-3-642-64326-2 e-ISBN-13: 978-3-642-60264-1
DOI: 10.1007/978-3-642-60264-1

Softcover reprint of the hardcover 1st edition 1998

Typesetting (Data conversion) : Zechnersche Buchdruckerei, Speyer

SPIN: 10558429 19/3133-5 4 3 2 1 0 – Printed on acid-free paper

Preface

The manuscripts in this book were generated from a conference occurring at the University of Heidelberg in September 1996. These manuscripts have been reviewed and updated by the designated authors in late 1997 for publication in early 1998.

Conferences occur for a variety of reasons. These include the need to exchange information where complex activities are undergoing reassessment or change. For the emergency and critical care management of stroke this is certainly the situation. Today, both the primary care and the neurologic physician must provide medical care in an environment where daily change in the knowledge base of: brain function, disease mechanism(s), therapeutic efficacy, and cost control are all occurring. In addition, patient advocacy has become increasingly complex because government, employers, insurers, health care providers as well as families all desire a voice in the physician relationship with the patient. Our conference subject was the organization of rapid care delivery and the development of a rational basis for treatment of a previously untreatable disorder acute stroke. Thus, the obvious need for multiple open and free discussions about priority setting and modification of current treatment plans. Clearly, the face to face opportunities provided by this first conference on Emergency Management And Critical Care Of Stroke (EMACCOS) are required when patient care issues are as complex as these.

Neuroscience is new to the experience of active therapeutic intervention. We would argue that the prior absence of therapeutic imperative in neurology was welcomed as a fortunate convenience by many physicians. However, times have changed. Now, for acute neurologic disorders it is clear that the era of contemplative diagnosis and indirect consultative care is ended. In the case of physicians who provide the principal care for stroke victims, this is particularly true. As scientists studying brain injury we have known for several decades that the time dependence of the threshold for producing acute brain injury places rigid constraints on the opportunities to reverse any acute brain disorders, particularly stroke. With the advent of a successful clinical trial of t-PA for acute ischemic stroke this time dependence of medical intervention becomes a primary priority in a way that is novel for the majority of physicians. For these reasons the principles that have governed the time dependent delivery of care in our emergency rooms and intensive care units are finally being adapted to the requirements of acute stroke care. We wish to share the experiences of a large group of physicians and scientists who have been preparing for this era of acute intervention.

The EMACCOS conference represents the first attempt to share the wisdom of acute care researchers from neurology, neurosurgery, neuroradiology and basic science for the benefit of the stroke victim. The epidemiology of stroke is compelling. With an annual incidence of over 150 events per 100 000 population, a significant association of age and stroke events, as well as the prolongation of life expectancies throughout the world the importance of stroke will not go away for the foreseeable future. When the disease process produces one of the highest levels of dependency of any modern disease the economic impact is unquestionable. Thus the cost of acute care represents only the beginning of an even larger burden for society when stroke occurs. Estimates of the hospital costs for stroke vary significantly over the range of $ 10 000 (TIA) to $ 40 000 (SAH) depending on the exact diagnostic grouping and medical care system. Economic dependence after the occurrence of stroke is an even larger cost with estimates in the range of 10 to 20 billion dollars for the United States alone. Both the sufferings of the victims and the economic burden for our society are independently justification enough for investment in a major educational and research effort to improve our medical care system for stroke. This conference began to address that educational need.

Stroke occurs in many different forms requiring individualized approaches. This book addresses both the hemorrhagic and the ischemic forms of the disease. The precise needs for each disease such as: aneurysmal subarachnoid hemorrhage, arteriovenous malformation, anterior and posterior circulation ischemic infarctions are different. These specific needs are provided by many different types of physicians. In order to address the entire set of stroke care needs we have designed a multispeciality conference that includes the perspective of neurologic surgeons, radiologists, anesthesiologists, scientists and principal care physicians from the emergency, intensive care and neurologic departments. We hope we have presented the perspectives of the entire set of physician care givers who will interact with the stroke patient during the acute portion of the patient's illness. It was our goal to develop an open forum where the exchange of clinical research from each of these areas can occur. We believe that he "vertical integration" of efficient and effective patient care for the stroke victim can be promoted amongst the entire group of medical professionals and developed into a better organized, more socially beneficial effort. There are no "final answers" in stroke care now. The current clinical trials represent only small improvements in the outcome of selected groups of stroke patients. We do not fully understand: how to select patients for differing types of treatment, how to prevent complications of treatment, or which new techniques developed for one stroke problem are applicable to other stroke subtypes as well. These qualifications are no more obvious than in the area of acute ischemic stroke where we observe the most exciting about recent advances. Treating stroke in the first 3 hours after occurrence requires explicit organization of emergency services, radiology, neurology, and substantial support from nursing, surgery and hospital pharmacy.

Frequently concerns have been raised that patient selected constraints make thrombolytic treatment applicable to only a small number of all stroke victims. However it is possible to improve the size of the treatable group of patients to at least 28% if there is an optimized refferral system as recently shown by a research group from Cologne, Germany. Unfortunately, the patient benefits remain small in both numbers of victims experiencing reversal of symptoms and in the magnitude of improvement of these symptoms. By explicitly promoting discussion and self directed criticism of stroke care results from each of these stroke care delivery areas we hope to address these deficiencies and improve the overall results.

This book attempts to address all the obvious needs of our area: Improving patient education/awareness of stroke symptoms and treatments, emergent patient diagnosis and treatment, optimal patient selection, effective use of computed tomography, MRI and angiographic techniques, optimizing drug therapy, utilization of critical care techniques, overall organization of patient care and the prediction of clinical outcomes. To all of us who are spending our days with the stroke victim, it is clear that we can do more in the areas of protecting the brain from further damage, promoting recovery of specific neuronal circuits that might allow for the return of lost functions, and explicitly organizing goal directed care. If improvements in these areas can occur, then we will reduce the entire cost to society of stroke as an illness. With this book we have recorded our conference proceedings to introduce the first steps in the direction of stroke care improvement. We hope that many others will follow in an effort to serve better the unmet needs of our patients.

Heidelberg and Baltimore, April 1998

Thorsten Steiner
Werner Hacke
Daniel F. Hanley

Acknowledgement

An undertaking as large as the First Emergency Management and Critical Care of Stroke conference cannot be successfully performed without the assistance of a large number of individuals. It is only with the good will, voluntary effort and interest of these individuals that this conference was successfully held. No professional conference organization company was involved. Local events and conference arrangements were organized by Petra Gunter and Marion Wilczek with assistance from Jochen Pilz and Markus Winter. The conference proceedings were audiotaped and photographed by Markus Winter and Anja Anzer. These audiotapes were organized and transcribed by Janis Kelly, Tammy Brown and Theresa Alt.

The conference was supported by:
Research Group of Neurologic Intensive Care; World Federal of Neurology (WFN); European Federation of Neurological Sciences (EFNS); Arbeitsgemeinschaft für Neurologische Intensivmedizin (ANIM) der Deutschen Gesellschaft für Neurologie (DGN); Section Critical Care Neurology, American Academy of Neurology (AAN).

Financial Sponsorship for this conference was provided by Boehringer Ingelheim. This allowed for the concept of EMACCOS to be presented and developed without the advocacy of Boehringer Ingelheim no conference would have occurred. Additional initial support was provided by Glaxo Wellcome (Bad Oldesloe/Germany, Uxbridge/UK); Janssen-Cilaq (Neuss/Germany and Beerse/Belgium); Sanofi (München/Germany); Baxter (Round Lake, IL).

Other contributors included:
Bayer (Leverkusen/Germany); Cerebro Vascular Advances, Inc (San Antonio, TX); CIBA-Geigy (Frankfurt/Germany); Fresenius (Bad Homburg/Germany); Grünenthal (Stolberg/Germany); Hoechst (Bad Soden/Germany).

The production of the proceedings by Springer Publishers, Berlin–Heidelberg–New York, has been made possible by a special educational grant of Lilly Inc., Indianapolis, IN and Hoechst-Marion Roussel, Kansas City, KS.

Table of Contents

List of Contributors

Alfred Aschoff
Department of Neurosurgery
Im Neuenheimer Feld 400
69120 Heidelberg, Germany

Jean-Claude Baron
INSERM Unité 320
Centre Cyceron
Boulevard H. Becquerel B.P. 5229
14074 Caen, France

Amesh Bhardwaj
c/o Raymond C. Koehler
John Hopkins Hospital
Blalock 1404
Baltimore, MD 21287, USA

T. P. Bleck
Department of Neurology
University of Virginia
Health Sciences Center
School of Medicine,
Box 394
Charlottesville, VA 22908, USA

Cecil Borel
Department of Anesthesiology
Box 3094
Duke University, Medical Center
Room 3413-D, Duke Hospital North
Durham, NC 27710, USA

Gudrun Boysen
Hvidovre Hospital
Department of Neurology
30 Kettegaard Alle
2650 Hvidovre, Denmark

Joseph P. Broderick
University of Cincinnati
Department of Neurology 231
Bethesda Ave. 4010 MSB
Cincinnati, OH 45267–0525, USA

Thomas Brott
Stroke Research
University of Cincinnati
Medical Center
231 Bethesda Avenue
RM 4010 MSB
Cincinnati, OH 45267–0525, USA

Guy L. Clifton
University of Texas
Houston Medical School
Department of Neurosurgery
6431 Fannin Street
Suite 7.148
Houston, TX 77030, USA

Steven Davis
The Royal Melbourne Hospital
Department of Neurology
Melbourne, Victoria 3050
Australia

Hans-Christoph Diener
Direktor der Neurologischen
Universitätsklinik
Hufelandstrasse 55
45122 Essen, Germany

Michael Diringer
Washington University
Department of Neurology
McMillian 401
Box 8111
660 South Euclid
St. Louis, MO 63110, USA

Geoff A. Donnan
Austin & Repatriation
Medical Center
Department of Neurology
Studley Road
Melbourne, Victoria 3084,
Australia

John M. Eskridge
Department of Neurosurgery
RI-20 University of Washington
School of Medicine
1959 N.E. Pacific Street, Box 356570
Seattle, WA 98195, USA

Cesare Fieschi
Università degli Studi di roma
"La Sapienza"
Dipartimento di Scienze Neurologiche
I Cattedra di Clinica Neurologica
Vialle dell'Università, 30
00185 Roma, Italia

James M. Findlay
Neurosurgical Associates
HYS Centre, Suite 500
11010–101 Street
Edmonton, Alberta, Canada

Matthew Fink
Department of Neurology
Beth Israel Medical Center
317 E 17th Street
New York, NY 10003, USA

Marc Fisher
Memorial Health Care
Department of Neurology
119 Belmont Street
Worcester, MA 01605, USA

James C. Grotta
Department of Neurology
University of Texas Medical School
6431 Fannin #7044
Houston, TX 77030, USA

Ulrich Grzyska
Neurologische Universitätsklinik
Abt. Neuroradiologie
Martinistrasse 52
20246 Hamburg, Germany

Georg Hamann
Department of Neurology
Ludwig-Maximilian University
Marchioninistrasse 15
83177 München, Germany

Mary Fran Hazinski
School Safety Project Coordinator
Vanderbilt University
243 Medical Center South
2100 Pierce Ave.
Nashville, TN 37212, USA

Michael Hennerici
Klinikum Mannheim
Neurologische Klinik
Theodor-Kutzer-Ufer
68167 Mannheim, Germany

Hans Hennes
Department of Anesthesiology
Johannes Gutenberg University
Langenbeckstrasse 1
55131 Mainz, Germany

Randolph Higashida
UCSF Med. Ctr.
505 Parnassus Ave., L–352
San Francisco, CA 94143–0628, USA

Higashi Hondo
Department of Neurological Surgery
School of Medicine
The University of Tokushima
Kuramoto 3–18–15
Tokushima 770, Japan

U. M. Illievich
c/o C. K. Spiss
Department of Anesthesiology
and General Intensive Care
University of Vienna
General Hospital
18–20 Währinger Gürtel
Vienna 1090, Austria

Otto Kempski
Institut für Neurochirurgische
Pathophysiologie
Postfach
55101 Mainz, Germany

J. R. Kirsch
c/o Raymond C. Koehler
John Hopkins Hospital
Blalock 1404
Baltimore, MD 21287, USA

Raymond C. Koehler
John Hopkins Hospital
Blalock 1404
Baltimore, MD 21287, USA

Dietrich Kühne
Abt. Röntgendiagnostik
und Neuroradiologie
Alfried Krupp Krankenhaus
Alfried Krupp Strasse 21
45117 Essen-Rüttenscheid, Germany

Rüdiger von Kummer
Department of Neuroradiology
Universität of Dresden
Fetscherstrasse 74
01307 Dresden, Germany

Richard E. Latchaw
Department of Radiology
PO Box 016960 (R-109)
Miami, FL 33101, USA

John R. Marler
Division of Stroke and Trauma, NINDS
Federal Building, Room 800
7550 Wisconsin Avenue
Bethesda, MD 20892, USA

Etsuro Mori
Gyogo Brain and Health Center
Neurology Service
520 Saisho-Ko
Himeji 670, Japan

Erich Rickels
Neurochirurgische Universitätsklinik
Medizinische Hochschule Hannover
Konstanty-Gutschow-Strasse 8
30625 Hannover, Germany

E. Bernd Ringelstein
Westfälische Wilhelms-Universität
Klinik und Poliklinik für Neurologie
Albert-Schweitzer-Str. 33
48129 Münster, Germany

M. Shibuya
Chukyo Hospital
Minami-ku
Nagoya 457-8510, Japan

T. Shimizu
Cerebrovascular Division
Department of Medicine
National Cardiovascular Center
5-3-7, Fujishiro-dai, Suita
Osaka 565, Japan

Claus K. Spiss
Department of Anesthesiology and General Intensive Care
University of Vienna
General Hospital
18-20 Währinger Gürtel
Vienna 1090, Austria

Thorsten Steiner
Universität Heidelberg
Neurologische Klinik
Im Neuenheimer Feld 400
69120 Heidelberg, Germany

H. Takahashi
c/o Raymond C. Koehler
John Hopkins Hospital
Blalock 1404
Baltimore, MD 21287, USA

James C. Torner
University of Iowa
Department of Preventive Medicine & Environmental Health
2811 B Sleinler Bldg.
Iowa City, IA 52242-1008, USA

Richard J. Traystman
Department of Anesthesiology/Critical Care Medicine
The Johns Hopkins University School of Medicine
600 North Wolfe Street
Blalock 1408
Baltimore, MD 21287, USA

Stanley Tuhrim
Department of Neurology
Clinical Program in Cerebrovascular Disease
The Mount Sinai Medical Center
Box 1137
One Gustave L. Levy Place
New York, NY 10029-6574, USA

Andreas Unterberg
Neurochirurgische Universitätsklinik
Klinikum Virchow
Krankenhaus Berlin UKRV
Augustenburger Platz
13353 Berlin, Germany

Daniel A. Wecht
University of New Mexico Hospital
2211 Lomas Boulevard NE
Albuquerque, NM 87106, USA

Justin Zivin
Department of Neurosciences 0624
UCSD School of Medicine
9500 Gilman Drive
La Jolla, CA 92093-0624, USA

Improving Early Referral and Emergency Care in Acute Stroke

J. P. Broderick, H.-C. Diener, E. Mori, E. Rickels, and M. F. Hazinski

Introduction

Tissue plasminogen activator (TPA) and other new drugs that may improve outcome if acute stroke is treated early, but optimal use of these agents will require earlier stroke detection by the public, faster transportation of the stroke patient to the hospital, faster evaluation by emergency room staff, and prompt administration of therapeutic agents. Improving stroke referral and treatment systems is key to achieving maximum benefits from these new agents.

Organizing a Better Patient Referral System

J. Broderick

Effective therapy requires early arrival of the patient at the hospital. This, in turn, requires early recognition by patient and family that a stroke may be happening. No matter how good treatment is, it will be useless if given too late. However, a community survey in the United States revealed that only 27% of the public could name even one warning sign of stroke [1]. When asked, respondents were likely to mention dizziness and headaches as warning signs.

Once stroke is suspected, the next requirement is for immediate contacting of emergency medical service and prompt transport to the hospital. This requires that emergency medical services approach the stroke patient like a trauma patient, with the assumption that "every second counts" and the designation of stroke as a Level One emergency like heart attack or severe trauma (Fig. 1).

Optimal care requires emergency department evaluation and treatment by a stroke team incorporating the emergency department, radiology, pharmacy, and the clinical laboratory. The key role on this team is a physician experienced at treating stroke.

The main obstacles to be overcome in emergency care of stroke are thus patient recognition of stroke, patient access to the hospital, patient evaluation in the hospital, and obtaining treatment by an experienced physician. The referral network for handling cases of suspected stroke can be a major resource for overcoming these obstacles.

One such network has been set up in Cincinnati, Ohio. This network includes 19 hospitals in an area of 1.3 million people. It is tied together by an excellent emergency transportation network. Ambulance personnel and paramedics are

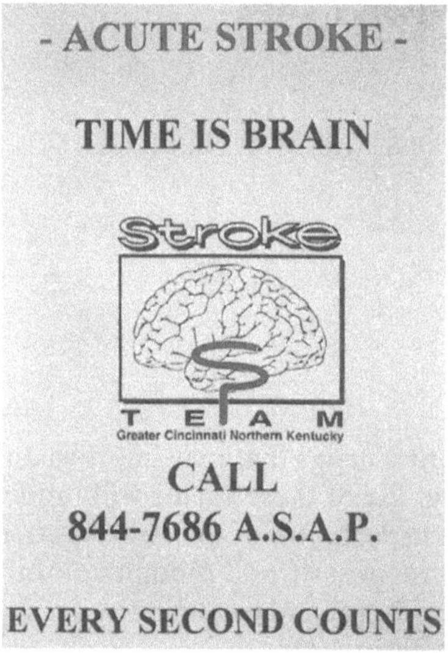
- ACUTE STROKE -
TIME IS BRAIN
Stroke
T E A M
Greater Cincinnati Northern Kentucky
CALL
844-7686 A.S.A.P.
EVERY SECOND COUNTS

Fig. 1. Time is Brain

considered to be part of stroke team and are given continuing medical education about stroke. The network of contacts and relationships also includes hospitals, physicians, nursing homes, emergency departments, and clinics.

Time to emergency department arrival is largely determined by where the patient calls for help. A pilot study in Cincinnati, Charlottesville, Virginia, and Cornell University Hospital in New York City found that those who called the "911" emergency number available in most U.S. cities got to the hospital nearly twice as fast as those calling their physician or the hospital itself (Fig. 2). Mean minutes between initial medical contact and emergency department arrival were 155 for those calling emergency services, 379 for those calling a private physician, and 333 for those calling the hospital [2].

A subsequent study in Cincinnati found that once the call came to the emergency medical service number, the time spent was 3 minutes from dispatch to arrival at the patient, 22 minutes to evaluate at the scene, and 17 minutes to travel to

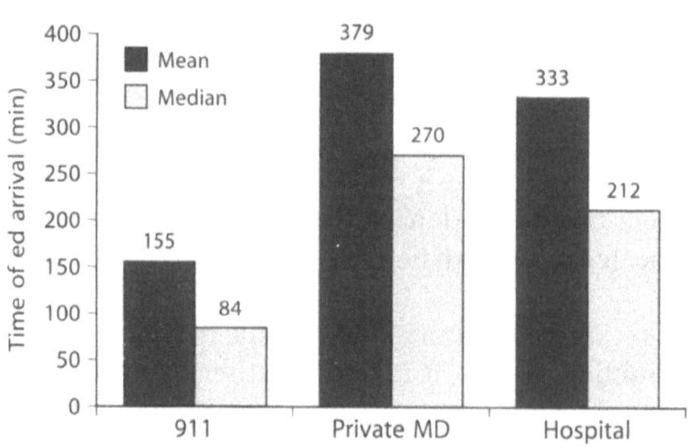

Fig. 2. Initial Medical Contact Versus Time of ED Arrival

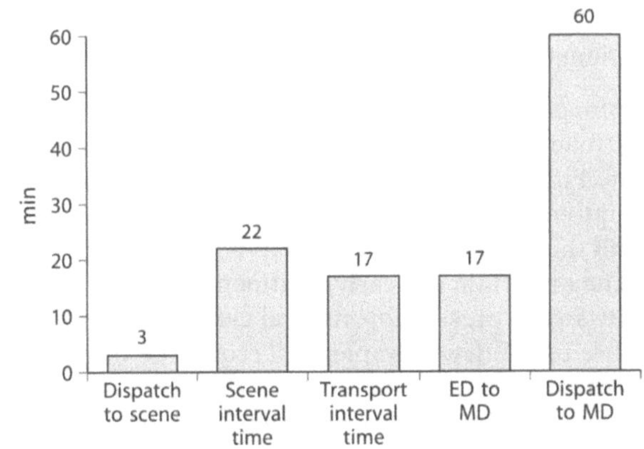

Fig. 3. Prehospital Time Intervals

the hospital (total 40–45 minutes) [3] (Fig. 3). One correctable problem this study identified was that emergency service dispatchers often did not tell the ambulance team that a possible stroke was involved. This suggests that more attention should be given to educating dispatchers on the signs of possible stroke.

This study also found that it took as long for the patient to see at physician once at the hospital (17 minutes) as to be transported from home to the hospital. Another 42 minutes passed after that, while the patient waited to get a computed tomography (CT) scan (Fig. 4). These times can be significantly reduced if a trained, coordinated stroke team is in place.

Two initiatives which would improve the time to treatment would be to follow U. S. National Stroke Association guidelines for assessing all departments and setting up protocols for evaluation and treatment [4], and to set up needed stroke team services by telephone while en route to the hospital. The coordinated stroke referral system often works best when implemented by an interested, experienced physician and an experienced nurse coordinator.

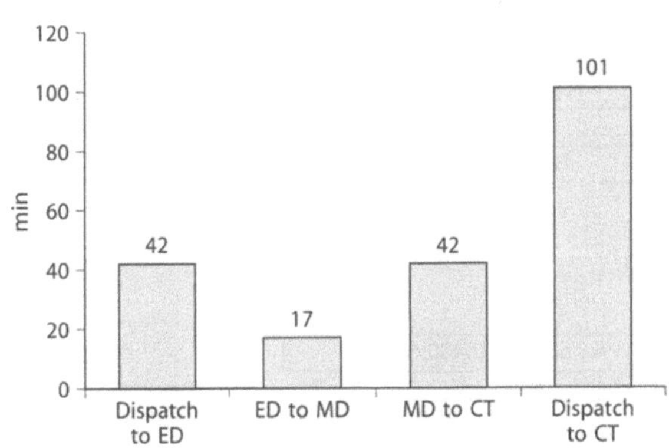

Fig. 4. Emergency Department Time Intervals

Teaching the Public About Stroke

C. Diener

Approaches to the problem of improving general public recognition of the signs of stroke must vary somewhat depending on country, but some aspect are common. First is the need to provide information to help the public recognize the symptoms of stroke. Use of a new term like "brain attack" may help people understand that a stroke is as urgent as a "heart attack" or myocardial infarction.

The importance of early treatment must be stressed. Only 42% of patients with acute stroke present for medical care within 24 hours of symptom onset [5]. Effective use of new therapies will require getting the patient to the hospital within 60–90 minutes of onset. There is evidence from the U.S. that an effective public education campaign can decrease the median time to hospital arrival from 3.2 hours to 1.5 hours [6]. A similar study from Germany found that a public education campaign reduced the median admission delay from 8 to 5 hours [7]. Education campaigns should be primarily directed at people at high-risk of stroke.

The aim of public education initiatives is to teach people to recognize the symptoms of stroke, to realize that urgent medical attention is needed, to use the emergency transportation service, and to go to the correct hospital. Media tactics include radio and television interviews, newspaper articles written by stroke specialists, lectures at primary care centers, lectures at emergency departments, and mailings.

Stroke Referral in Japan

E. Mori

Japan has a similar emergency referral system linking primary care clinics, secondary emergency hospitals, and higher emergency medical centers (Fig. 5). The referral system working well for ischemic heart disease and hemorrhagic stroke but less well for ischemic stroke. The Japanese population numbers 120 million, and there are a total of 60,000 rescue service workers and registered emergency

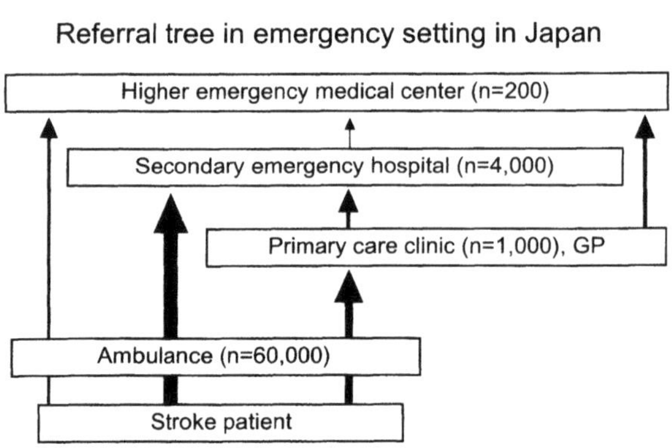

Fig. 5. Referral Tree in Emergency Setting in Japan

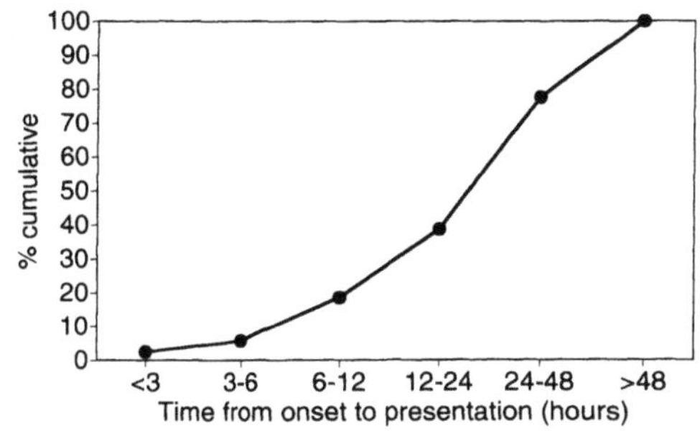

Fig. 6. Time from Onset to Presentation

care specialists, all of whom belong to the fire department. The number of board-certified neurologists is 3,000, which contrasts with the greater number of neurosurgeons or cardiologists. There are about 1,000 primary care clinics, 4,000 secondary emergency hospitals, and 200 higher emergency centers. There are also about 12,000 CTs and 2,400 MRIs.

Less than 10% of patients with ischemic stroke present for medical care within 6 hours after symptom onset, although virtually all patients are transported to the hospital within 40 minutes after the call for emergency services is made (Fig. 6). About 80% of patients present within two days after onset. The stapes of diagnosis and triage are working well for hemorrhage but not as efficiently for ischemic stroke. The secondary emergency hospitals are primarily involved in the treatment of acute ischemic stroke. Their capability to manage acute ischemic stroke patients is limited. It would be difficult for them to make a very early specific diagnosis and triage, and they would be reluctant to refer their patients very early to higher facilities. There is little awareness of the need for urgent treatment of ischemic stroke. The development of an established specific treatment for ischemic stroke would allay this situation.

The main problem in Japan, as elsewhere, is the lack of public awareness of the signs of stroke and the need for urgent treatment. In addition, there is a shortage of neurologists to cover emergency ischemic stroke cases. However, this will be gradually overcome since the number of neurologists is increasing by 200 per year. Meanwhile, the key to improving stroke care would appear to be how secondary emergency hospitals are assigned in the scheme of emergency stroke treatment.

Modern Communications Technology

E. Rickels

One possibility for providing more access to stroke specialists, improving patient care, reducing the need for transport, and reducing costs is through video teleconferencing. This approach is being used in Germany with considerable success.

Each year there are about 340,000 head injuries. Neurosurgical facilities in Germany include 4933 beds in neurosurgical departments and 578 beds in neurosurgical intensive care units (ICUs). Fewer than 10% of these beds are available for emergencies. This bed shortage leads to a frequent need to transport patients. Specialty centers accept all patients but the sending hospital must accept patient return at any time, even if the patient has been sent directly from the operating room. The goal of this system is to accept only patients who need neurosurgical therapy, and for shortest possible time.

This raises three problems for specialists at the specialty centers. The first is how to communicate with outside doctors about emergencies. The second is how to discuss the patient being operated and transferred back to the sending hospital. This includes such things as managing the return after surgery, conferences for after care, and follow-up CT scans. The third problem is how to accept only patients who need neurosurgery.

The solution to the communications and resource problems has been intensive consultation using video teleconferencing systems to analyze magnetic resonance (MR), CT, and x-rays images before transfer to decide whether operation is needed or not. The system permits eye-to-eye contact between doctors at different sites had has been well accepted in all participating hospitals.

The system is now handling over 300 cases per year, including head injuries, intracerebral hemorrhages, cerebral tumors, spinal lesions, and hydrocephalus. Before telecommunication CT/MR scans were sent by taxi for a neurosurgical assessment, or the patient was transported by helicopter or ambulance, and often sent back without surgery. Now 67% of the presented cases are found not to need neurosurgical intervention, at a saving of about 1,600,000 DM/year. The cost of the video teleconferencing equipment is 50,000–115,000 DM.

The Role of Emergency Personnel

M. F. Hazinski

In order to preserve maximum neurologic function following stroke, effective stabilization and treatment of the stroke patient must be accomplished within a few hours. The entire medical system which the patient encounters must operate at maximum efficiency to enable the use of potential therapies within the window of opportunity available. In the 1970s trauma surgeons first focused attention on the emergency medical services system in the U.S. because they determined that about 25 percent of trauma deaths could be prevented if emergency medical services were improved [8].

In the 1980s emergency medical services and pre-hospital care were further refined by advances made in the detection and treatment of myocardial infarction. Defibrillation was added to pre-hospital care, leading to the steps of assessment and stabilization with the ability to quickly diagnose and treat arrhythmias, particularly with defibrillation [9].

Greater emphasis on early assessment of possible stroke has increased the importance of prompt stabilization and treatment of the patient. The American Heart Association has developed guidelines and algorithms which highlight the central aspects of pre-hospital and emergency care for patients with cardiovascular emergencies, which now include stroke. In the United States this creates a standard of care which has some legal implications. Most importantly, all paramedics are required to complete advanced cardiac life support (ACLS) training [10]. The American Heart Association has worked with, for example, the European Resuscitation Council, the Resuscitation Council, of Australia, and the Resuscitation council of Southern Africa to promote these guidelines.

The National Heart Attack Alert Program identified four keys to management of the heart attack. These are known as the "four D's" [11]:

- the patient's arrival at the Door of the emergency department
- the patient's Data are gathered
- the Decision to treat and how to treat is made Drug therapy is used.

Three more D's can be considered in the patient with a brain attack or stroke [12]:

- Detection,
- Dispatch (activation of emergency medical service system personnel)
- Delivery via emergency medical service alerting, identification, and transport of the patient.

The "window of opportunity" for treatment often referred to as "Time is brain." [13]. The pressure to act within that window has increased performance requirements for emergency personnel, both in the ambulance and in the emergency room. Half of stroke patients in the U.S. use the emergency medical services (EMS) system [2, 14]. The mean time between symptom onset and the EMS call is 2.6 h. In contrast, patients who are brought in by their families have a delay of over 5 hours [15]. A public education campaign in Houston succeeded in reducing the interval from onset of symptoms to presentation in the emergency department from more than 19 hours to an average of two hours [16].

One reason for delay is that EMS dispatchers and personnel sometimes do not identify stroke symptoms. An unpublished study from the University of Cincinnati found that EMS personnel correctly identified actual strokes only 72.1% of the time, and incorrectly identified non-strokes as strokes in 27.9% of cases. Prevention of delays will require education of EMS dispatchers, education of paramedics and emergency medical technicians, development of simplified assessment tools, streamlining of scene protocols, and consistent pre-arrival notification of hospital.

A paramedic quick screen for stroke should include identification of focal neurologic symptoms, determining if there is a well-established onset, and noting if the patient is aged 18–80 [14]. The information from this screen should be called in to the emergency department to trigger activation of the stroke team. Further useful information can be obtained using a modified stroke scale rather than the Glasgow Coma scale. Determine facial palsy by asking the patient to smile. Determine bets motor arm by asking the patient to hold arms up. Determine language problems (aphasia, dysarthria) by asking the patient to repeat phrases [17].

Delays at the hospital can occur as a result of inadequate communication from the field, inappropriate triage and prioritization, and inadequate or unreliable neurologic examination. This can be prevented by giving stroke patients high priority in triage, streamlining protocols and checklists, and having standing orders for emergency management of stroke so evaluation and care are not delayed until arrival of consultant. Consequently, education must target triage nurses and physicians, and people who will first encounter the patient in the emergency department, who must perform standardized stroke scale evaluations.

Unnecessary studies and tests should be prevented. Often an ER doctor or local physician in a primary clinic will perform multiple studies to "make sure the patient has a stroke" before activating the stroke system or neurology consult. A big delay, often 2 or more hours, occurs before the performance of the CT scan. To shorten the time until the patient gets to CT, the first physician to see the patient should have the authority to order the CT scan. Finally, the emergency department should maintain a streamlined checklist for eligibility for thrombolytic therapy. A sample checklist of yes and no items for eligibility of thrombolytic therapy might have the following structure (adapted from [18]:

"Yes" Checklist (required)
- Oriented, can cooperate, appropriate
- Signs consistent with anterior, lacunar, or posterior infarct (or partial MCA)
- CT scan complete and interpreted
- Within 3 h of onset of symptoms
- Age 18–80 years
- BP: 60–185 mmHg/less than 110 mmHg

"No" Checklist (exclusionary)
- No cerebrovascular hemorrhage on CT
- No major infarction, hypodensity
- No seizure
- No rapidly improving NIHSS
- No previous intracranial hemorrhage
- No recent major surgery or head trauma
- No BP over 185/110 mmHg

Delays can be prevented by the development of timed, streamlined protocols, called "Code Stroke" or "Brain Attack Alert," with limited diagnostic studies. this requires that the neurologist and primary physician become very familiar with ER protocols and that everyone work together to ensure completion of these protocols within designated time targets. There also should be 24-hour CT availability with a third or fourth generation CT, and priority use so the stroke patient does not wait in the hallway behind every possible trauma victim.

Conclusion

Studies on emergency management of stroke in several countries indicate a near-universal problem with delayed detection of possible stroke and extended times between symptom onset and presentation of the patient for emergency medical treatment. Multi-step campaigns to educate the public about to identify the signs of stroke are needed. The importance of the 6-hour "window of opportunity" for treatment also means that efficient referral networks and faster communication between medical personnel must be adopted, perhaps using telecommunication systems. Finally, the considerable delays that occur after the patient is in the emergency room point up the need for streamlined system, perhaps including assembling a stroke team to deal with "brain attacks" in the emergency setting as well as reexamining standard procedures and reducing the use of unnecessary tests.

References

1. Pancioli A, Broderick J, Kothari R, et al (1997) Public perception of stroke warning signs and potential risk factors. Stroke 28:236–238
2. Barsan WG, Brott TG, Broderick JP, et al (1993) Time of hospital presentation in patients with acute stroke. Arch Intern Med 153:2558–2566
3. Kothari R, Barsan W, Brott T et al (1995) The potential prehospital care providers to impact early treatment in acute stroke: a pilot study. Stroke 26:937–941
4. Houser G, Spilker J (1995) The NSA clinical trials acceleration program (CTAP). Presented at a meeting on Ischemic Stroke: Recent Advances in Understanding and Therapy, International Business Communications, South Burham, MA, pp 107-143
5. Albers MF, Bartels C, Dawson DV (1990) An analysis of time of presentation after stroke. JAMA 263:65–68
6. Barsan WG, Brott TG, Olinger CP, et al (1988) Identification and entry of the patient with acute cerebral infarction. Ann Emer Med 17(11):1192–1195
7. Muffelmann B, Glahn J, Kunz S, et al (1995) Busse: Strategien zur fruhen Aufnahme von Schlaganfallpatienten. Nervenarzt 66:111–115
8. Trunkey DD (1982) The value of trauma centers. ACS Bulletin 67:5–7
9. Cummins RO, Graves JR, Horan S, et al (1984) The relative contributions of early defibrillation and aces interventions to resuscitation and survival from prehospital cardiac arrest. Ann Emerg Med 18:468–469 (Abst)
10. Cummins RO (ed) (1997) Textbook of advanced cardiac life support. The American Heart Association, Dallas
11. National Heart Attack Alert Program Coordinating Committee, 60 Minutes to Treatment Working Group (1994) Emergency department: rapid identification and treatment of patients with acute myocardial infarction. Ann Emer Med 23:311–329
12. Hazinski MF (1996) Demystifying the recognition and management of stroke. Currents in Emergency Cardiac Care 7:8
13. Gomez J (1993) Editorial: Time is Brain. J Stroke Cardiovascular Disease 3:1–2
14. Lyden PD, Rapp K, Babcock T, et al (1994) Ultrarapid identification, triage, and enrollment of stroke patients into clinical trials. J Stroke Cerebrovascular Dis 4:106–107
15. Kothari R, Barsan W, Brott T, et al (1995 Jun) Frequency and accuracy of prehospital diagnosis of acute stroke. Stroke 26(6):937–941
16. Bratina P, Greenberg L, Pasteur W et al (1995) Current emergency department management of stroke. Stroke 26:409–414
17. Kothari R, Hall K, Broderick J, et al (1997) Early stroke recognition, developing an out of hospital stroke scale, (WHAT) Nead Emerg Med. In press
18. Cummins RO (ed) Acute stroke. In: Textbook of advanced cardiac life support. American Heart Association, Dallas, pp 10–16

Referral Patterns in Clinical Trials

S. Davis and G. Donnan

Introduction

The characteristics of patients studied in clinical trials are important because of effects on the accuracy of trial results and because of implications for application of new therapies outside the research setting. Experience also indicates that the existence of a well-publicized acute stroke clinical trial can improve referral patterns and bring patients into the hospital more quickly due to improved education of physicians and the general public about the benefits of early intervention.

How Many Patients Fit Into the Time Window?

Potential time treatment windows for interventional stroke strategies directed at acute tissue rescue (Table 1) remain somewhat uncertain. Recombinant tissue plasminogen activator (rTPA) is effective within 3 hours [1] and may have a longer time window in patients without major ischemia on acute computed tomographic (CT) scan [2]. The time windows for most neuroprotective agents are unknown, although many trials are using a 6-hour timeframe. Treatment times are similarly uncertain for antithrombotic therapies, particular with low-molecular-weight heparin and heparinoids. Treatment with these agents may be possible up to 24–48 hours after stroke.

This extended time may be due to the ischemic penumbra, the area where the brain tissue is hypoperfused but metabolically still viable [3] (Fig. 1). There is some evidence to suggest that parts of the ischemic penumbra are salvageable for as long as 24 hours after stroke. Timing of intervention is critical, and certainly the expectation now is that emergency transport and treatment are essential.

The problem areas in management of acute ischemic stroke are delays in emergency transport and delays in the emergency department. The nihilistic attitudes towards stroke sometimes encountered reflect a lack of perceived effective treatment and are in contrast with rapid arrival at the emergency room after myocardial infarction or severe trauma. The clinical effect is undeniable. Even in patients arriving acutely, few will be eligible for stroke trials. In one study only 5–10% of patients arriving within 6 hours of symptom onset were eligible for the clinical trial [4]. Suggested remedies include direct triage to a stroke unit, recruiting emergency room physicians as trial co-investigators, linking reimbursement to

Table 1. Experimental strategies for acute tissue rescue

Reperfusion therapies	Neuroprotective therapies
• Thrombolysis	• Calcium channel antagonists
- Intra-arterial	- Nimodipine
- Intravenous rTPA	• NMDA receptor antagonists
• Hemodilutional therapy	- Cerestat
- Isovolemic	- Magnesium
- Hypoverlemic	- Selfotel
• Antithrombotic therapies	• Glutamate release inhibitors
- Heparin	- Lubeluzole
- Low-molecular-weight heparinoids	• Free radical scavengers
- Aspirin	- Lazaroids
• Miscellaneous	• Miscellaneous agents
- Pentoxifyline	- Glycine polyamine antagonists
- Prostacyclin	- Sodium channel blockers
- Ancrod	- Neurotrophic factors

the interval from stroke onset, and having a neurologist based in the emergency department.

Clinical investigators worldwide are also facing a new problem: attempts to abolish surrogate trial consent. Most countries currently allow consent by next of kin for patients with depressed conscious state or dysphasia. This particularly affects patients with acute ischemic stroke. This procedure is now under threat in many countries, and new restrictions require that only the patient or an appointed guardian can consent. We have certainly had the situation of trying to contact guardians at 3:00 in the morning for some studies, and it is difficult to accomplish. If this requirement becomes widespread, it is predicted to reduce stroke trial accruals by 33% [5]. It will particularly affect the entry of patients with severe, language impairing strokes into clinical studies.

Previous studies have found that stroke type can affect hospital arrival time, and particularly that patients with hemorrhagic stroke are likely to arrive earlier [6–8]. Involvement of primary care practitioners is likely to delay arrival [7]. Older patients may arrive earlier, as do those who have strokes in the morning, particularly at work [4]. Barsan et al. also found that patients arrive earlier if the emergency services number is the first one called [9].

Data from several stroke studies also suggest that a stroke clinical trial itself can improve the arrival hospital times of stroke patients, apparently due to increased awareness on the part of the general public as well as of the participating clinical staff. The National Institutes of Health (NIH) pilot study of rTPA found increased use of the 911 emergency number and improved stroke arrival times, apparently due to public and professional education campaigns [10]. Lyden et al. reported an increase from 0.4 to 0.7 patients per month who arrived at the hospital within 3 hours of stroke onset, due to the institution of a stroke hotline, urgent 911 number, use of the "paramedic quick screen" assessment tool, training of personnel, and use of an in-hospital "code stroke" [11].

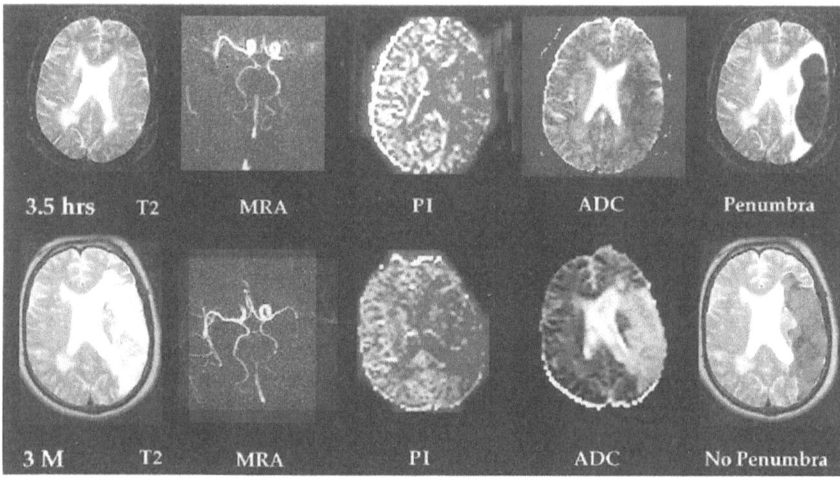

Fig. 1. This illustrative case demonstrates the ischaemic penumbra. This patient had a large left middle cerebral artery infarct. The upper panel indicates studies performed at three and a half hours after stroke onset. The T2 - weighted MR scan is normal with a lack of flow in the left middle cerebral artery on magnetic resonance angiography. Acute perfusion (PI), diffusion (ADC) mismatch is evident, with a larger perfusion abnormality (blue) and the penumbra (yellow) is the mismatch between these parameters. The outcome studies at three months show expansion of the ischaemic infarct core into the penumbral region with a large infarct at outcome and poor functional state

Researchers at the Royal Melbourne Hospital (Melbourne, Australia) reviewed a consecutive series of stroke patients who presented over a 6-month period. Of the 163 consecutive stroke patients, 79% were infarcts and 22% were hemorrhages. All patients were screened for the interval between symptom onset and hospital arrival time. About 40% of patients arrived within 6 hours (Fig. 2). Ambulance arrivals were a median of 4.0 hours after onset; arrivals by other means were a mean of 19.0 hours ($p<0.001$). Older patients arrived somewhat earlier than younger ones, but there was no influence of stroke type or gender on arrival time.

Applying the eligibility criteria of the NIH rTPA trial, and additionally excluding patients with major ischemic changes on the sub-3 hour CT scan, the RMH study showed that only about 12% of patients presenting within 180 minutes of symptom onset would be eligible for rTPA (Table 2). Applying the eligibility of other clinical trials, the RMH study found that only 11% of patients would be eligible for a neuroprotective trial (Pharmacia-Upjohn TESS II Tirilazad trial) and 15% of patients would be eligible for a low molecular weight Heparin Trial (Sanofi Winthrop Fis bis Fraxiparine Trial). Thus, even with early arrival times, in terms of acute stroke trials, few patients remain eligible. This may change as more effective therapies are identified and a wider proportion of patients become eligible for acute therapy.

Rapid recognition and ambulance transport remain the most important factors for increasing accrual in trials of acute stroke interventions. Organizational strategies are crucial, including facilitating emergency department triage, insti-

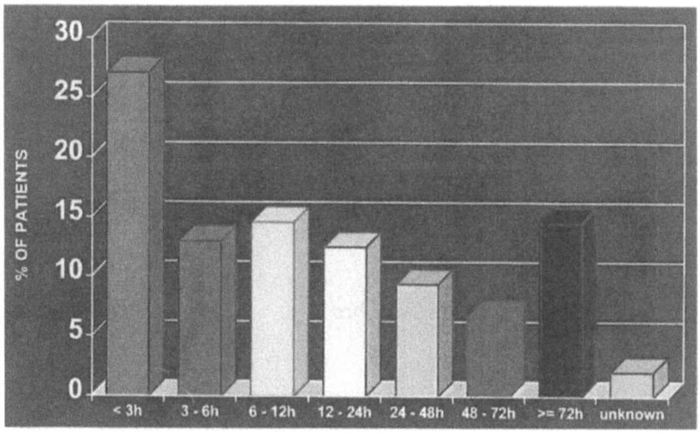

Fig. 2. Arrival Delay for Ex-Hospital Stroke Patients

tuting ethically sound simplified consent procedures, and setting up acute stroke units in hospitals.

Characteristics of Patients in Early Treatment Trials

Two important questions in designing and evaluating clinical trials are, "What is the hypothesis to be tested?" and "What is the nature of the population base?" The Northeast Melbourne Stroke Incidence Study (NEMESIS) was launched to capture accurate data on stroke incidence in the community. A further trial of the posterior circulation only (Australian Urokinase Stroke Trial - AUST) has been commenced with a lomg 24-hour time window (Fig. 3). This patient population is less common (as evidenced from the NEMESIS Study) but represents an important group because of poor prognosis when vessel obstruction is shown on angiography. The goal was to examine the impact of new therapies at the community level. The population includes about 303,000 patients with an expected 1500 strokes per year. Early data on 79 patients showed that the most common

Table 2. Acute stroke data (patients admitted December 1995 – 31 May 1996 with ischemic stroke). 0–3 hours trial exclusion based on NIH tPA trial, ECASS CT criteria

Abnormal CT scan (evidence of early major infarction)	3/33*	10%
Prothrombin time >15 seconds	6/33	18%
No deficit measurable on NIH scale (or rapidly resolving)	7/33	21%
Severe deficit	6/33	18%
Seizure with stroke onset	1/33	3%
Patient requiring anticoagulation	1/33	3%
Pre-existing confounding deficit/recent stroke	3/33	10%
Total eligible	**4/33**	**12%**

* i.e. 3% of RMH ischemic stroke patients

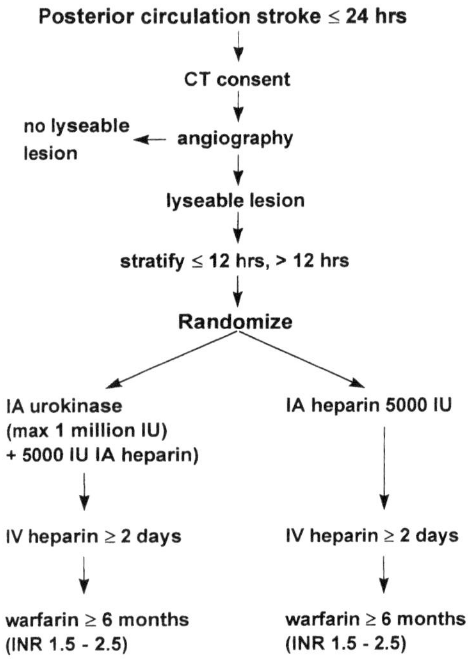

Fig. 3. AUST Protocol

stroke subtype was partial anterior cerebral ischemia (PACI, 33%), followed by posterior cerebral ischemia (POCI, 16%), total anterior cerebral ischemia (TACI, 14%), and lacunar cerebral ischemia (LACI, 14%).

Patients with partial anterior ischemic stroke or lacunar stroke were most delayed in arriving at the hospital (Mean of 8 and 12 hours after symptom onset, respectively.)

Clinical trials in different countries have reported quite different rates of stroke subtypes among their patient populations. The ASK (Australian Streptokinase) trial had 88.2% hemispheric stroke, 4.4% lacunar stroke, 5.9% brainstem stroke, and 1.5% unknown subtype [12]. The MAST-I (Multicenter Acute Stroke Trial – Italy) trial had 68% non-lacunar stroke and 32% lacunar stroke [13]. Finally, The NINDS (National Institute of Neurological Disorders and Stroke) trial had 11% small vessel occlusive, 44.8% cardioembolic, 41.6% large vessel occlusive, and 2.6% other types of stroke.

Conclusion

The potential treatment window for acute stroke is thought to be about 6 hours in most cases. With some neuroprotective agents this may extend to 24 hours, due to the possibility of rescuing ischemic but still viable penumbral tissue around the core lesion. Data from clinical trials suggest that there may be significant differences in the types of stroke which present for treatment, and that the delay before hospital arrival may be affected by a variety of factors such as age and stroke type. One fact is clear across all countries, disease types, and population subgroups, however: The vast majority of patients with strokes do not arrive at the hospital soon enough to benefit from the new thrombolytic or neuroprotective treatments. This problem can be improved at least somewhat by aggressive education campaigns directed at the general public and at physicians in the referral area.

References

1. The National Institute of Neurological Disorders and Stroke rt-PA Stroke Study Group. (1995 Dec 14) Tissue plasminogen activator for acute ischemic stroke. New Eng J Med 333(24): 1581–1587
2. Hacke W, Kaste M, Fieschi C, et al (1995 Oct 4) Intravenous thrombolysis with recombinant tissue plasminogen activator for acute hemispheric stroke. The European Cooperative Acute Stroke Study. JAMA 274(13): 1017–1025
3. Warach S, Dashe JF, Edelman RR (1996 Jan) Clinical outcome in ischemic stroke predicted by early diffusion-weighted and perfusion magnetic resonance imaging: a preliminary analysis. J Cerebral Blood Flow & Metabolism 16(1): 53–59
4. Herderschee D, Limburg M, Hijdra A, et al (1991) Timing of hospital admission in a prospective series of stroke patients. Cerebrovasc Dis 1: 165–167
5. Saver JL, Starkman S, Fox S, et al (1995) The impact upon clinical stroke trials of restricting informed consent. Stroke 26: 157 (Abst)
6. Kay R, Woo J, Poon WS (1992) Hospital arrival time after onset of stroke. J Neurol, Neurosurg & Psych 55(10): 973–974
7. Rosen DM (1993) New directions for acute stroke therapy. Med J Australia 158(2): 78–80
8. Alberts MJ, Bertels C, Dawson DV (1990) An analysis of time of presentation after stroke. JAMA 263(1): 65–68
9. Barsan WG, Brott TG, Broderick JP, et al (1993) Time of hospital presentation in patients with acute stroke. Arch Intern Med 153: 2558–2561
10. Barsan WG, Brott TG, Broderick JP, et al (1994) Urgent therapy for acute stroke. Effects of a stroke trial on untreated patients. Stroke 25: 2132–2137
11. Lyden PD, Rapp K, Babcock T, et al (1994) Ultra-rapid identification, triage and enrollment of stroke patients into clinical trials. J Stroke Cerebrovasc Dis 4:106–113
12. Donnan GA, Davis SM, Chambers BR, et al (1996 Sep 25) Streptokinase for acute ischemic stroke with relationship to time of administration: Australian Streptokinase (ASK) Trial Study Group. JAMA 276(12): 961–966
13. Anonymous (1995 Dec 9) Randomised controlled trial of streptokinase, aspirin, and combination of both in treatment of acute ischaemic stroke. Multicentre Acute Stroke Trial–Italy (MAST-I) Group. Lancet 346(8989): 1509–1514

Pathophysiology of Stroke

M. Diringer and O. Kempski

Introduction

Distrubed regulation of cerebral blood flow (CBF), inadequate oxygen delivery, and elevated intracranial pressure all contribute to damage of ischemic stroke. Each of these areas offers a target for intervention in emergency care of stroke. Work examining the interactions between cerebral blood flow, oxygen delivery, brain metabolism, and neuronal injury suggest that there may be better ways to predict the risk of neuronal damage and protect brain tissue. Studies of the mechanisms causing increased intracranial pressure have identified a number of mediators which may become therapeutic targets. These areas are examples of the key role played by basic research into physiological phenomena in our efforts to improve the outcome of ischemic stroke.

Pathophysiology of Severe Vascular Brain Injury

Regulation of cerebral blood flow (CBF) is influenced by pressure autoregulation, oxygen delivery, flow-metabolism coupling, the influence of arterial carbon dioxide pressure ($PaCO_2$) on cerebrospinal fluid (CSF) pH and blood viscosity. Positron emission tomography (PET) scanning is useful for examining these interactions and defining ischemia in acute brain insults.

CBF and brain metabolism are closely coupled. In the idealized autoregulation curve, blood flow remains constant over a wide range of perfusion pressures due to changes in cerebrovascular resistance (Fig. 1). As perfusion pressure decreases vessels dilate, resistance goes down, and flow is maintained. When vessels can no longer dilate CBF falls. Chronic hypertension shifts this curve to the right, which becomes an important issue in treating blood pressure in hypertensive patients. As the oxygen content of arterial blood falls, cerebral blood flow must rise to maintain constant oxygen delivery.

The primary source of energy for the brain is oxidative metabolism of glucose. There is no significant storage of substrate in the brain, which is why a brief interruption of the blood supply can result in energy failure. Since CBF is tightly coupled to metabolism stimuli that increase metabolism will cause a secondary increase in CBF and vice versa.

A useful tool for assessing the relationship between CBF and metabolism in head injury is the arteriovenous difference in O_2 content ($A\text{-}VDO_2 = CaO_2 - CvO_2$).

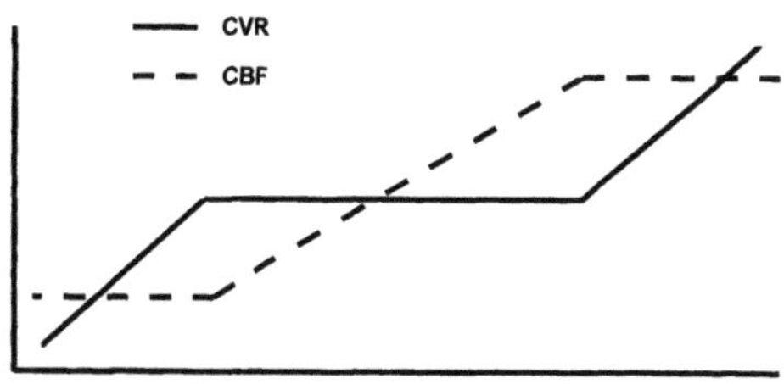

Fig. 1. Idealized relationship between cerebral perfusion pressure (CPP) and cerebral blood flow (CBF). Across a wide range of CPP (defined as mean arterial pressure – intracranial pressure) CBF remain constant (autoregulation). This occurs as a result of increases (as CPP rises) or decreases (as CPP falls) in cerebrovascular resistance (CVR). The changes in resistance are due to dilation or contraction of small penetrating arterioles. Once the ability of these vessels to dilate or contract is exceeded (upper and lower limits of autoregulation) CBF becomes pressure passive

Oxygen content is $CaO_2 = 1.34 \times ([Hg] \times O_2\ sat) \times (PaO_2 \times 0.003$. The value for arterial O_2 content is 18–20 vol % with normal hematocrit. If the patient has suffered a large blood loss, hematocrit may be low and therefore arterial oxygen content may be low. The brain removes is about 1/3 to 1/2 of the delivered O_2 under normal resting conditions, leaving a substantial reserve. The normal range of difference between arterial and venous oxygen content (A-VDO_2) is 4.5 to 9.0 vol % [1].

There are two main ways of assessing the relationship between CBF and metabolism in patients. One can perform global measurement with the jugular bulb catheter, which is inserted into the jugular vein, advanced to the jugular bulb, and used to sample global cerebral venous blood. However, in brain insults which have a focal area of dysfunction such as intracerebral hemorrhage (ICH), contusion, or subdural hematoma, jugular catheters may not detect important focal areas of increased O_2 extractions. PET scanning is useful in these settings because it can measure the regional relationship between CBF and metabolism.

Traditionally ischemia is defined as CBF below approximately 20 ml/100 g/min [2]. In acute vessel occlusion the CBF falls dramatically. In an attempt to maintain a constant metabolic rate, the oxygen extraction fraction rises. Once it is maximal, if the CBF rises any further, the cerebral metabolic rate begins to fall and remains low. If perfusion is re-established there is a hyperemic response, in which the blood flow is quite high, metabolism is low, so the oxygen extraction fraction falls very low (Fig. 2). This period is sometimes referred to as "luxury perfusion." In the chronic state metabolism remains low, CBF decreases, the two are matched, and oxygen extraction fraction is normal.

If there is a primary reduction in metabolism, this definition of ischemia must be modified. When the metabolic rate is suppressed, a CBF which would otherwise produce neurologic symptoms and neuronal death can be tolerated. For example, pre-treatment with barbiturates can protect against reduced CBF [3]. When there is a primary reduction in metabolism, the fall in CBF is secondary to reduced metabolism, and O_2 extraction fraction and A-VDO_2 are normal or reduced.

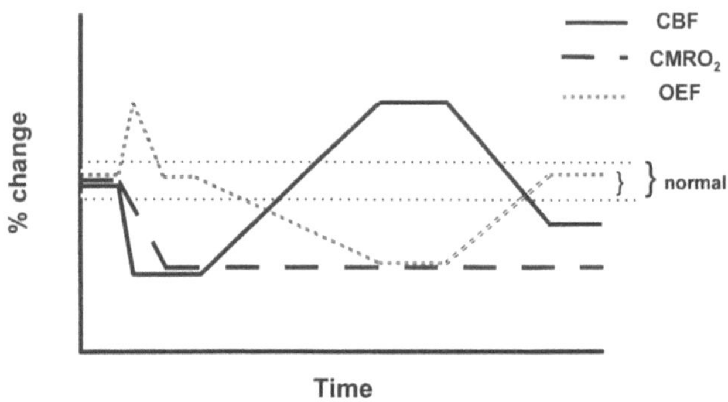

Fig. 2. Cerebrovascular changes in ischemic infarction. Idealized representation of changes in cerebral blood flow (CBF), cerebral metabolic rate for oxygen ($CMRO_2$) and oxygen extraction fraction (OEF) following vessel occlusion. Initially CBF falls and OEF rises in an attempt to meet metabolic needs. Since oxygen delivery is inadequate $CMRO_2$ falls. Once cell death and reperfusion have occurred CBF rises to above normal levels (hyperemia or luxury perfusion). $CMRO_2$ remains low since the tissue is dead. Since flow exceedes metabolic needs OEF is low. Over time CBF falls to below normal levels and metabolic rate remains low. Since flow and metabolism are both reduced OEF returns to normal levels

To summarize, under normal conditions with normal CBF and normal metabolic rate, O_2 extraction fraction remains normal. When there is a primary reduction in metabolic rate, CBF falls as well, but again O_2 extraction fraction remains normal. If there is an increase in the metabolic rate, as occurs in hyperpyrexia or seizures, again O_2 extraction remains normal. If there is a primary reduction in blood flow, metabolism remains normal and the oxygen extraction fraction begins to rise. This is sometimes referred to as "misery perfusion," when CBF is just adequate to maintain normal neuronal function.

If CBF drops further and the O_2 extraction fraction is maximal, ischemic injury occurs. In the late phase where "luxury perfusion" occurs the CBF is elevated out of proportion to metabolism, and the O_2 extraction fraction is very low.

The critical factor for the tissue's ability to produce high-energy phosphates, maintain membrane integrity, and neuronal function, is the tissue pO_2 rather than the difference between the arterial and venous oxygen content. Therefore, the magnitude of the rise in O_2 extraction fraction or A-VDO_2 may not be the best indicator of the effect on tissue oxygenation. This is especially important when there are variations in arterial oxygen content. Defining ischemia in terms of cerebral venous oxygen content (CvO_2) may be useful in defining ischemia in stroke, in vasospasm following subarachnoid hemorrhage, intracerebral hemorrhage and traumatic brain injury.

Injury in ICH occurs via several mechanisms. These include direct tissue disruption from hematoma, re-bleeding, edema, and possibly ischemia. Hypertension is common following ICH and may contribute to rebleeding and the development of cerebral edema. However, hypertension also may be helpful by protecting against ischemia. The clinical dilemma is whether to lower the blood pressure to reduce risks or not lower it to protect against ischemia.

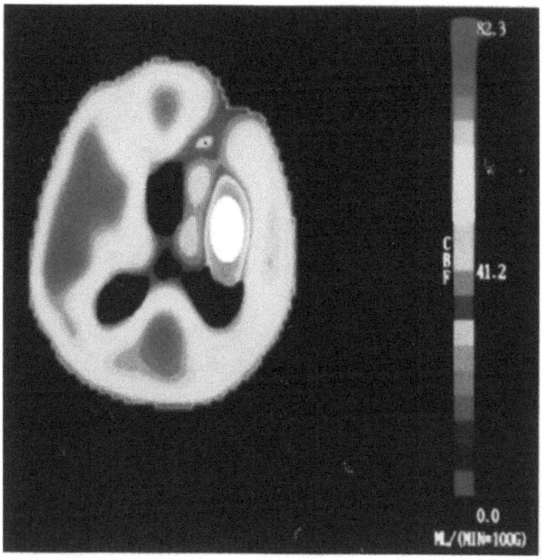

Fig. 3. Cerebral blood flow following acute intracerebral hemorrhage. This figure of a typical basal ganglion hemorrhage shows the CT scan superimposed on the PET image. The white area defines the limits of the hematoma. The blue region surrounding it shows the area of reduced blood flow

In a case of typical basal ganglion hemorrhage with CT scan superimposed on the PET image, a region around the hematoma shows a reduction in blood flow. Comparison of CT and PET images with regard to oxygen extraction fraction reveals that a patient with a relatively small hemorrhage may have significantly areas of increased oxygen extraction (Fig. 3). Conversely, a patient with a much larger hemorrhage may have only a relatively small area of increased oxygen extraction (Fig. 4).

Biology of Elevated ICP: Vasogenic and Cytotoxic Edema

The causes of intracranial pressure (ICP) elevation include head injury, ischemia, hypoxia, intracranial hemorrhage, tumors, hydrocephalus, abscesses, infections, and encephalopathies. The most important factor is brain edema, of which there are two subtypes: vasogenic and cytotoxic.

The most important consequence of elevated ICP is herniation. A more common result is a reduced perfusion pressure and secondary ischemia. Compliance is an important factor in this situation. Compliance of the brain means that subsequent additions to the intracranial volume will produce greater increases in ICP (Fig. 5). The more volume added to the intracranial compartment, the greater the likelihood of a steep increase in ICP.

In the upper range of ICP A-waves and B-waves may be encountered (Fig. 6). A-waves are 2- to 15-minutes of steep ICP increases occasionally to 80 mmHg, which are then followed by a sudden decrease to only slightly elevated levels. B-waves are small waves of 10- to 30 mmHg at a frequency of one to two per minute.

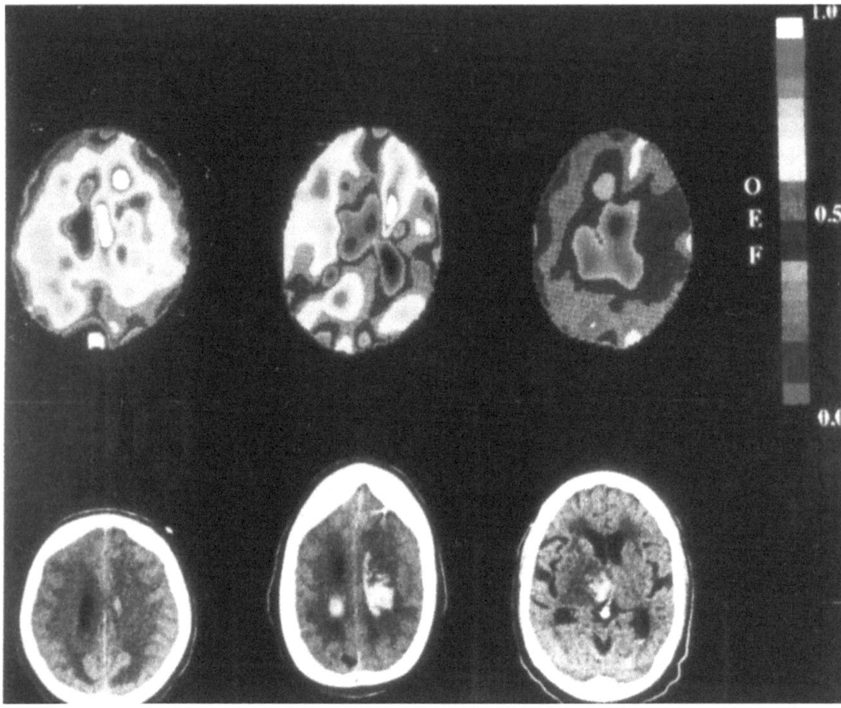

Fig. 4. Hemorrhage size and oxygen extraction fraction. A range of changes on oxygen extraction fraction can be observed in intracerebral hemorrhage. In the patient at left, the CT scan (bottom left) shows a fairly small hemorrhage, but the PET image (top left) shows two significant regions of increased oxygen extraction. The patient at center has a larger hemorrhage as demonstrated on CT scan (bottom center), but PET image shows little increased oxygen extraction fraction (top center). The patient at right has a moderate-sized hematoma (bottom right) but with no elevation in oxygen extraction (top right)

Cerebral perfusion pressure (CPP) determines how much blood reaches the parenchyma. In considering reducing arterial pressure or controlling ICP, we must keep in mind that both these parameters determine perfusion pressure. First measure ICP if possible, then determine the perfusion pressure. A low CPP may cause secondary ischemia.

We have repeated Cushing's experiments in elevated ICP. We used 9 rabbits with chloralose anesthesia. First we introduced a gradual ICP increase by intraventricular CSF infusion, to an ICP of 50 mmHg. This was maintained for 10 minutes. Then a fast ICP increase was induced to a cerebral perfusion pressure of zero, which initiated the Cushing response. We monitored the parietal cortical microcirculation by laser Doppler scanning and the basilar artery velocity by transcranial Doppler. In addition, we monitored ICP, arterial pressure, and somatosensory evoked potentials. We found that over a wide range of cerebral perfusion pressures, the microcirculation does not change much, as would be expected due to autoregulation. We observed reduced flow in the micro-

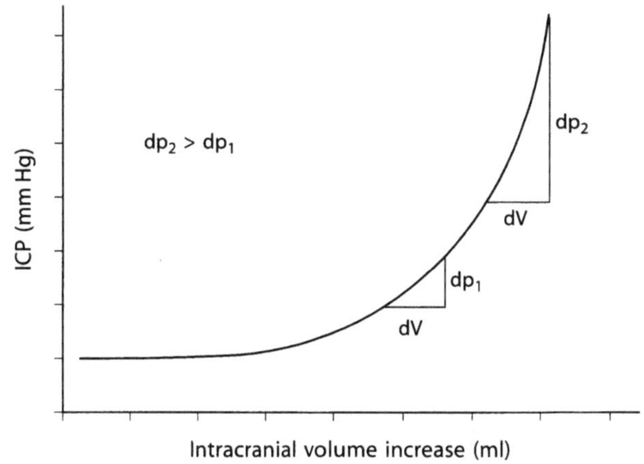

Fig. 5. Compliance of the brain. Subsequent additions to intracranial volume produce steeper changes in intracranial pressure

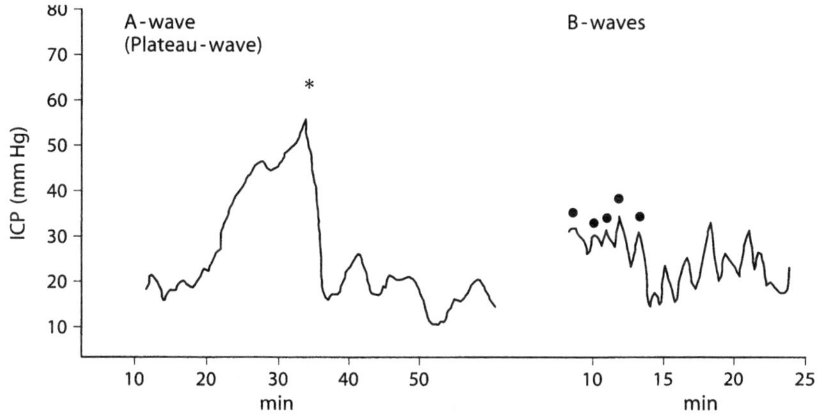

Fig. 6. A-waves and B-waves. These occur at higher ICP levels. A waves are 2- to 15-minute, steep ICP increases to 80 mmHg, followed by steep declines. B-waves are small 10–30-mmHg waves that occur at a frequency of one or two per minute

circulation only after the cerebral perfusion pressure dropped below 40 mmHg [4].

Large vessel velocity changed rather linearly with cerebral perfusion pressure. This can be seen clearly by calculating the resistance index flow velocity

$$RI = (FVs - FVd)/FVs$$

This is the systolic flow velocity (FVs) minus the diastolic flow velocity (FVd) divided by the systolic flow velocity (FVs). There is a strong linear relationship between the resistance index and cerebral perfusion pressure.

Combining the laser Doppler values with the resistance index demonstrated that the resistance index must be above 0.8 before there is a reduction of velocity in the microcirculation. Resistances in this range indicate that the perfusion of the parenchyma is at risk. Vasogenic edema is due to damage to the blood-brain-barrier, which leads to an influx of protein-rich plasma ultrafiltrate into the cerebral parenchyma. Due to the protein-rich edema fluid; brain water content increases. The plasma constituents, which under physiological circumstances are excluded from the brain, may interact with glia and neurons. Vasogenic edema is mediated by the kallikrein-kinin system, arachidonic acid and its metabolites (eicosanoids, free radicals), biogenic amines, cytokines, and thrombin [5].

Cytotoxic edema is due to intracellular water accumulation in the glia, neurons, and endothelial cells [6]. This is observed within minutes after interruption of the energy supply, as a swelling of cells and fluid consisting mostly of water and ions but no proteins. The consequences of cytotoxic edema are impaired cellular function and no reflow or low reflow because capillaries are compressed. This may provide benefits by sealing off damaged tissue and reducing blood-brain-barrier leakage in that vascular territory.

Four mediators of cytotoxic edema have been identified: acidosis, excitotoxins (glutamate), free fatty acids (arachidonic acid), and extracellular potassium over 15 millimoles. The first three of these mediators cause either dendritic swelling or nerve cell death. They all activate glial homeostatic mechanisms. Glial cells swell in order to clear these mediators from the extracellular space [7, 8]. This causes secondary elevation of ICP and sometimes secondary ischemia.

The process of vasogenic edema was demonstrated in a cat study by Baethmann et al. [9]. Cortical freezing was used to induce vasogenic edema. Edema fluid was sampled by nylon wick catheters to measure mediator substances. There were two experimental groups: one with sufficient CPP and one with critically low CPP. The researchers found that glutamic acid, an excitotoxin, was elevated in both groups. However, glutamate levels was significantly higher in the animals who had secondary ischemia after ICP elevation. These high levels of glutamate may cause further swelling of cells and thereby further damage ICP.

Identification of these mediators of both vasogenic and cytotoxic cerebral edema open the possibility of intervening to limit the damage associated with elevated ICP by modulating the concentration and/or activities of these substances. This may provide another neuroprotective strategy in the emergency care of stroke.

Conclusion

Advances in our understanding of the pathophysiology of ischemic stroke have revealed three areas which may be particularly promising for development of therapeutic interventions. Studies of the relation between inflammation and thrombosis point to the microvasculature as the primary target for neuroprotection. Studies of CBF and metabolism have identified areas in which intervention should be done cautiously and have provided a new tool, measurement of venous oxygen content, which may provide better clinical warning of impeding neuronal damage. The mediators of cytotoxic and vasogenic edema are appealing targets for preventing damaging elevations in ICP. All of these approaches offer the hope of intervening in the pathophysiologic processes that cause devastating long-term damage following stroke before such damage becomes irreversible.

References

1. Gibbs EL, Lennox WG, Nims LF, et al (1942) Arterial and cerebral venous blood arterial-venous differences in man. J Biol Chem 144:325
2. Astrup J, Symon L (1981) Thresholds in cerebral ischemia: the ischemia penumbra. Stroke 12:723–725
3. Hoff JT, Schmith AL, Hankinson HL et al (1975) Barbiturate protection from cerebral infarction. Stroke 6:28–33
4. Ungersbock K, Tenckhoff D, Heimann A, et al (1995) Transcranial Doppler and cortical microcirculation at increased intracranial pressure and during the Cushing response: an experimental study on rabbits. Neurosurgery 36:147–156; discussion 156–157
5. Wahl M, Unterberg A, Baethmann A, et al (1988) Mediators of blood-brain barrier dysfunctions and formation of vasogenic brain oedema. J Cerebral Blood Flow and Metabolism 8:621–634
6. Cohadon F (1987) Physiopathology of brain edema. Revue Neurologique 143(1):3–20
7. Kempski O, Staub F, Schneider GH, et al (1992) Swelling of C6 glioma cells and astrocytes from glutamate, high K concentrations or acidosis. In: ACH Yu, L Hertz, MD Norenberg, E Sykova, SG Waxman (eds) Progress in Brain Research Vol 94. Elsevier Science Publishers B.V., Elsevier, pp 60–75
8. Kempski O, Volk C (1994) Neuron-glial interaction during injury and edema of the CNS. Acta Neurochir [Suppl] 60:7–11
9. Baethmann A, Maier-Hauff K, Schurer L, et al (1989 Apr) Release of glutamate and of free fatty acids in vasogenic brain edema. J Neurosurgery 70(4):578–591

Autonomic Changes in Acute Cerebrovascular Disorders

C. Borel and G. Hamann

Many cerebrovascular disorders are associated with autonomic dysfunction, particularly subarachnoid hemorrhage (SAH), intracerebral hemorrhage (ICH) and ischemic stroke. The common basis for these problems is maximal activation of the sympathetic pathway, with parasympathetic coactivation. A major main clinical symptom is electrocardiograph (ECG) change that may include a long QT interval, torsades des points, ventricular arrhythmias (Fig. 1), and cerebral T waves. Cardiovascular changes include hypertension, tachycardia, or bradycardia. Neurogenic pulmonary edema may also occur, as well as metabolic changes in catabolism or sodiumpotassium function, and stress reactions such as agitation or anxiety which contribute to the risk of secondary rebleeding.

These autonomic disturbances are not only the result of a clinical complication but may also cause secondary clinical deterioration, initiating a vicious circle of pathophysiologic deterioration. For example, in ICH, the cerebral perfusion pressure may be reduced by the hemorrhage itself or by a rise in intracranial pressure. This leads to reduced tissue oxygen, and the end product is tissue damage (Fig. 2). Autonomic activation, mainly sympathetic stimulation, is a positive ef-

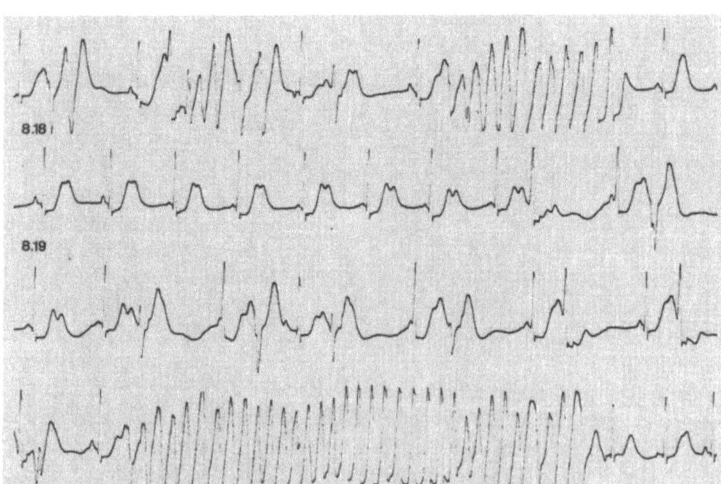

Fig. 1. Ventricular Fibrillation in Subarachnoid Hemorrhage. A major clinical symptom in acute stroke is electrocardiograph change, which may include ventricular arrhythmias

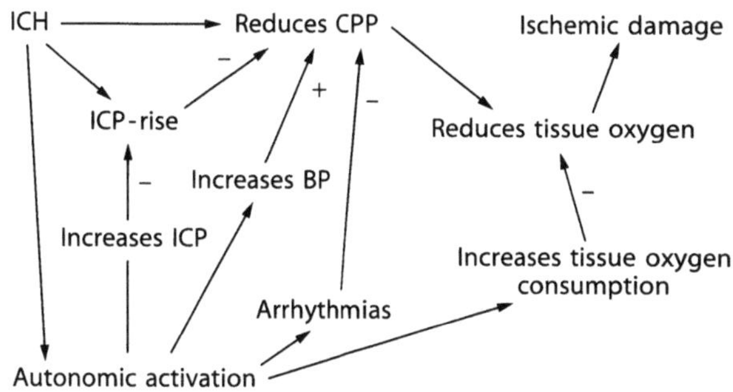

Fig. 2. ICH and Autonomic Activation. Autonomic disturbances are both the result of clinical complications and the cause of secondary clinical deterioration after acute stroke

fort to increase blood pressure, which may help maintain cerebral perfusion pressure, but sympathetic overstimulation and maximal increase in blood pressure can also increase intracranial pressure and damage the bloodbrain barrier.

The autonomic centers involved in cerebrovascular diseases are in the insular cortex, hypothalamus, periaqueductal gray matter, nucleus tractus solitarius, and nucleus ambiguous. Damage to these areas may be either direct or indirect. Damage to the dorsomedial or posterior hypothalamus causes sympathetic activation, whereas damage to the anterior hypothalamus causes vagal stimulation. The organization of these centers is best understood as a network of interactions. Direct damaging effects to the cerebral autonomic centers may be due to such events as vasospasm in the hypothalamic area in SAH. Secondary damage arises through more general mechanisms, most importantly ICP rise (especially in cases with transtentorial herniation) and global cerebral ischemia.

The role of intracranial pressure was established early in this century by Cushing [1]. The traumatic changes observed in animal studies indicated an acute, cranial, spaceoccupying lesion with sympathetic coactivation. Graf et al. demonstrated the role of sympathetic activation [2].

Hamann and colleagues continued this work in an investigation of 37 patients with SAH, 28 patients with spontaneous ICH, and 16 patients with acute ischemic stroke [3]. Daily blood samples were drawn and assayed for basic sympathetic activity (metanephrines and normetanephrines), peak sympathetic changes (epinephrine, norepinephrine, dopamine), and activity of the reninangiotensinaldosterone system (plasma renin activity, aldosterone).

In patients with SAH, normetanephrine, norepinephrine, aldosterone, and plasma renin activity were significantly elevated compared to a control group ($p < 0.01$). Twentyeight acute increases in the hormones were seen. Hormonal changes were caused by vasospasm ($n = 14$), rebleeding ($n = 7$), ICP rise ($n = 5$) or late hydrocephalus ($n = 2$). There was a positive correlation between the Gurusinghe Score, which measures thickness of the clot, and plasma renin activity ($r = 0.62$).

Similar changes were observed in the ICH patients. They had elevated norepinephrine, normetanephrine, and plasma renin compared to controls ($p < 0.05$). Twentyfour elevations of hormones were recorded, all in close timerelationship to ICP rises.

Patients who had large hemorrhage or who had hemorrhage with intraventricular bleeding had significantly higher plasma renin activity, normetanephrine, and norepinephrine activity. Patients who died also had significantly higher normetanephrine (1053 vs 316 micg/d, $p < 0.001$).

Patients with ischemic stroke displayed similar patterns. Mean plasma renin activity, normetanephrine, norepinephrine, and metanephrine were elevated compared to controls ($p < 0.05$). Sixteen elevations of the hormonal parameters were recorded, mainly for plasma renin activity, norepinephrine, and normetanephrine. In all cases an ICPrise was found to be the underlying mechanism. Patients who died had higher plasma renin activity and normetanephrine ($p < 0.01$).

Beta adrenergic blocking agents were tested because they have proven helpful in prevention of autonomic changes after severe head trauma [4]. SAH patients treated with intravenous metoprolol reduced the pulse rate and the need for antihypertensive agents. There was also a tendency toward better outcome in the treated group.

A wellknown and very typical part of the autonomic changes after stroke as well as any spaceoccupying intracranial disease is the neurogenic pulmonary edema. The second part of this chapter will address this model of an autonomic manifestation of central nervous system autonomic disorders.

Neurogenic Pulmonary Edema Following Stroke

Neurogenic pulmonary edema is a significant problem. It is associated with lesions to the hippocampus or medulla and thought to result from excess catecholamine release, which increases pulmonary capillary pressure, unbalancing the Starling equation and results in edema.

Respiratory care of stroke is a major source of cerebral protection. Respiratory management includes management of the airway and maintaining oxygenation. In many ways, cerebral protection is more dependent on respiratory care than on maintaining flow or preventing secondary injury. One of the main problems in stroke is how to assess and maintain the airway as the stroke evolves. Pulmonary edema contributes to those difficulties.

Neurogenic pulmonary edema (NPE) had been observed in a variety of neurologic disorders, particularly head trauma, intracranial hemorrhage, brain tumor, stroke, epileptic seizures, stellate and trigeminal nerve blocks, medullary lesions, meningitis, and polio. Data from Vietnam combat experience showed that soldiers with gunshot wounds to the head often died of NPE rather than gunshot wound, while soldiers with gunshot wounds to the spine did not develop NPE and were more likely to survive [5]. NPE can be caused experimentally by either penetrating or closed head wounds, and also by epidural lesions to the cranium, saline infusion, balloon expansion, lesions to the lower cervical spine, or bilateral cervical vagotomy [6].

The uniting feature of lesions associated with NPE is their localization in the hypothalamus or medulla (Fig. 3). These areas are responsible for autonomic

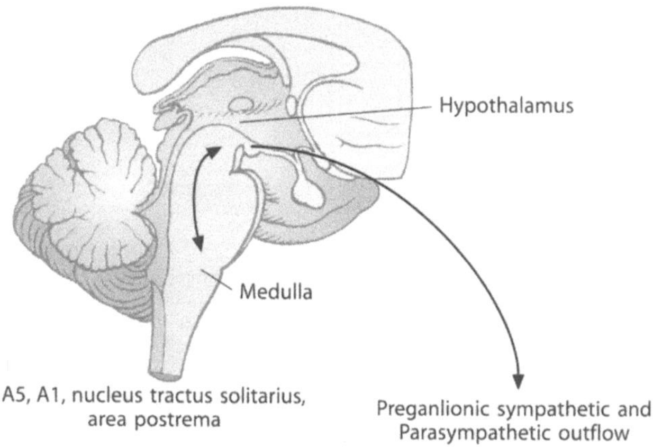

Fig. 3. Structures Mediating Neurogenic Pulmonary Edema. Lesions associated with neurogenic pulmonary edema are most commonly located in the hypothalamus or medulla

regulation. Injury to the hypothalamus may result in a massive outflow of preganglionic sympathetic and parasynpathetic catecholamines. Injury to the medulla may result in damage to the A5, A1, nucleus tractus solitarius, or area postrema.

The Starling equation tells us that flow across capillary is related to a constant which is multiplied by the hydrostatic pressure inside the capillary minus the hydrostatic pressure outside the capillary (Fig. 4a). The amount of flow across the capillary is usually determined by the hydrostatic pressure. There is normally a small flow into the interstitial space and then out through pulmonary lymph system. The interstitial space must be free of fluid if gas exchange is to occur and oxygen is to be taken up in the pulmonary venule.

A transient massive increase in pulmonary capillary pressure unbalances the Starling forces and can lead to acute pulmonary edema (Fig. 4b). This occurs because elevated hydrostatic pressure forces more fluid out of the capillary space and into the interstitial space, overwhelming the ability of the system to remove it and causing leakage into the alveolus (Fig. 4c).

Work by Malik et al. in anesthetized dogs demonstrated that pulmonary artery pressure and pulmonary perfusion pressure rises as a consequence of increased intracranial pressure (ICP) [7]. This study showed that pressures inside the pulmonary vascular system rise when ICP rises. This response includes an increase in pulmonary artery pressure, leftatrial pressure, and pulmonary perfusion pressure or pulmonary vascular resistance. Propranolol does not block this increase, but the alpha blocker phenoxybenzamine does.

Simon et al. demonstrated in anesthetized sheep that a seizure can cause pulmonary edema [8]. In this model seizures dramatically increased the aortic pressure. Furthermore, raising left atrial pressure with inflation of a balloon dramatically increased lung lymph flow, which forced fluid out of the capillary space and into the pulmonary interstitium (Fig. 5).

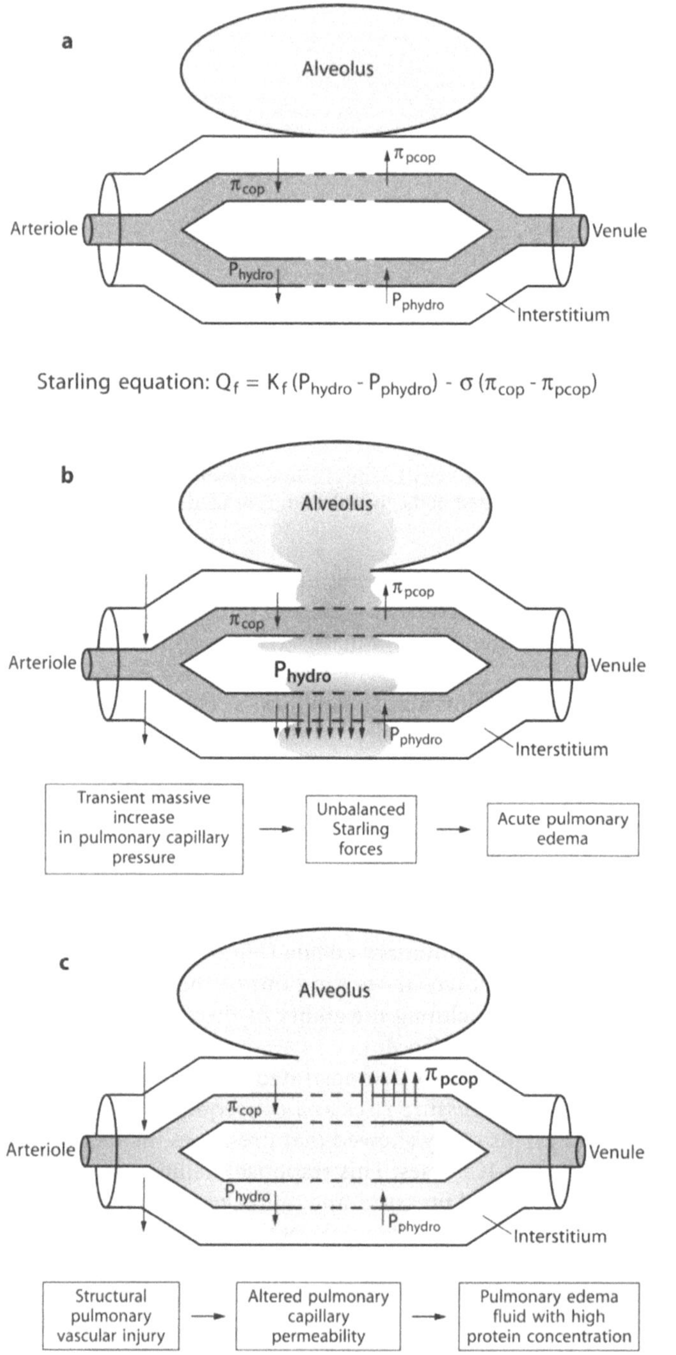
a
Alveolus
π pcop
π cop
Arteriole
Venule
P hydro
P phydro
Interstitium
Starling equation: Qf = Kf (Phydro - Pphydro) - σ (πcop - πpcop)
b
Alveolus
π pcop
π cop
Arteriole
P hydro
Venule
P phydro
Interstitium
Transient massive increase in pulmonary capillary pressure
Unbalanced Starling forces
Acute pulmonary edema
c
Alveolus
π pcop
π cop
Arteriole
Venule
P hydro
P phydro
Interstitium
Structural pulmonary vascular injury
Altered pulmonary capillary permeability
Pulmonary edema fluid with high protein concentration

Neurogenic Pulmonary Edema (NPE)

Diseases
- Head Trauma
- Intracranial hemorrhage
- Brain tumor
- Stroke
- Epileptic seizure
- Stellate and Trigeminal Nerve Block
- Medullary lesion
- Mennigitis
- Poliomyelitis

Experimental
- Head wound
  - penetrating
  - closed
- Epidural lesion
  - saline infusion
  - balloon expansion
- Lesion
  - hypothalamus
  - low c-spine
  - bilat. cervical vagotomy

Fig. 5. Causes of Neurogenic Pulmonary Edema. A number of disease states and experimental conditions are known to cause neurogenic pulmonary edema

Lymph plasma also increased, showing that plasma protein was being forced out of the capillary space and into the interstitium. The result was that raising left atrial pressure caused an increase in lung lymph flow and pulmonary edema. This implies that massive catecholamine release can cause pulmonary edema.

Another group of experiments suggested an alternative mechanism of pulmonary edema. In this model structural pulmonary vascular injury leads to altered pulmonary capillary permeability, causing fluid and protein leak into interstitial space and alveolus. In this model the hydrostatic pressures are fairly normal through the arterioles but there is massive leakage of protein across the capillary endothelial membrane into the interstitial space due to damage of the capillary endothelium. Leakage into the alveolus causes difficulties with gas exchange, and the leakage is so massive it cannot be overcome by interstitial clearance of osmotically rich pulmonary edema fluid.

McClellan et al. have published evidence supporting this possibility [9]. Work in anesthetized dogs showed that elevated ICP increases pulmonary vascular permeability to protein. The result was pulmonary edema associated with protein leakage.

There is evidence that this occurs in humans. Touho et al. examined NPE in the acute stage of hemorrhagic cerebrovascular disease [10]. This study included 38 patients with subarachnoid hemorrhage (SAH) or and intracerebral hemorrhage. Patients who developed NPE had: lower O_2 saturation, higher O_2 gradient across the pulmonary membrane, higher extravascular lung water, and pulmonary capillary leak occurring at lower capillary wedge pressures, rather than hydrostatic pulmonary edema. Patients in this study who developed pulmonary edema had very high extravascular lung water and very high alveolararterial oxygen differences, as compared to patients who did not develop pulmonary edema.

Fig. 4. **a** Starling Forces at the Pulmonary Capillary and Alveolar Junction. The balance of hydrostatic pressure (P) and osmotic pressure (σ) minimizes fluid leakage to the interstitial space. **b** Effect of Pulmonary Capillary Pressure. Transient increase in the pulmonary capillary pressure promotes leakage of fluid across the membrane resulting in classic "high pressure" pulmonary edema. **c** Importance of Capillary Membrane. Damage to the capillary membrane results in leakage of protein rich fluid across the membrane

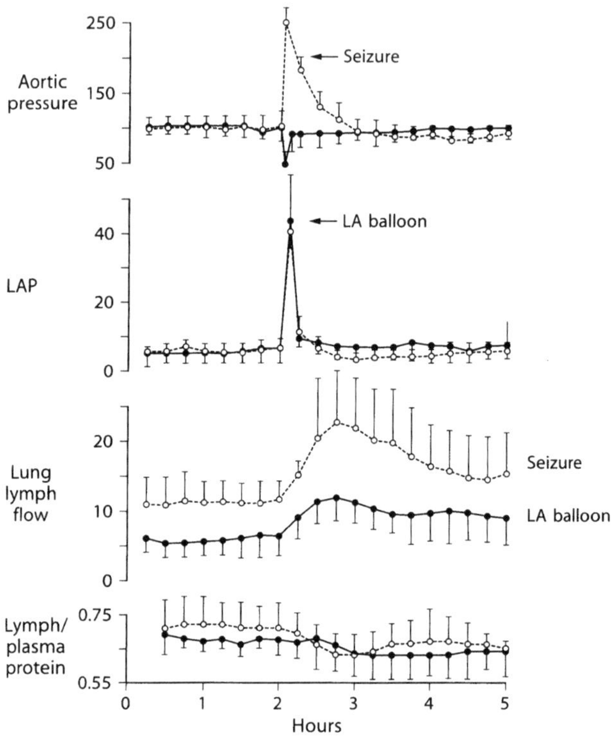

Fig. 6. Left Atrial Pressure and Lung Lymph Flow. Elevation of the left atrial pressure mimics the altered lung lymph flow observed in seizures. Either induced seizures or inflation of a left atrial balloon resulted in increasing lung lymph flow in an anesthetized sheep model. This indicates that seizures may cause pulmonary edema by elevating capillary hydrostatic pressure. (Reprinted with permission, Simon et al.) [4]

These data suggest that NPE does occur in patients with cerebrovascular disease and that it is associated with diffusion gradients for oxygen, not with high capillary wedge pressure. This is probably a capillary leakage phenomenon.

Clinically, NPE follows the rapid onset of neurologic injury, and there is an association with injuries that involve the hypothalamus (Fig. 6). NPE can be prevented or attenuated by alpha blockers and by central nervous system (CNS) depressants. Hemodynamic changes involve first an increased autonomic tone, then pulmonary edema with high protein content. Acute brain injury can disturb hypothalamic function, leading to a massive adrenergic discharge, pulmonary vasoconstriction, systemic vasoconstriction, increased pulmonary venous pressure, and a transient increase in pulmonary capillary wedge pressure. At the same time there is increased aortic and systemic arterial pressure, decreased leftventricular compliance, increased left atrial pressure and a shift of blood from the systemic to the pulmonary circulation, leading to pulmonary edema.

The massive increase in pulmonary capillary pressure unbalances the Starling forces and leads to acute pulmonary edema. Pulmonary hemorrhage can also occur. The clinical picture may include an early form of acute pulmonary edema in patients with seizures and massive adrenergic discharge during early intervention or when neurologic injury occurs.

NPE is sometimes seen in patients in interventional neuroradiology following disasters. On the other hand, patients admitted through the Emergency room who go through a delay before arriving at the intensive care unit develop pulmonary edema associated with a high protein concentration in a vascular leak phenomenon, which may occur somewhat later in the cascade of pulmonary injury.

Management requires heightening the index of suspicion that NPE may occur. An arterial line is indicated for patients at risk, such as those with autonomic instability or hypothalamic injury. Monitoring should include continuous oxygen saturation (pulse oximetry), a pulmonary artery catheter if the patient is hemodynamically unstable, and ICP monitoring if there is severe intracranial injury.

Supportive care should include supplemental oxygen, and often this is sufficient. Mechanical ventilation is sometimes needed in patients requiring pulmonary artery catheters or ICP monitoring. Positive endexpiratory pressure (PEEP) is the best way to treat low oxygenation when the alveoli become flooded.

Drug therapy has not yet been tested in humans. Possibilities include alpha adrenergic blockers such as phenoxybenzamine or labetalol. There may also be clinical benefit from calcium channel blockers such as nifedipine or nicardipine in reducing pulmonary vascular resistance. If the pulmonary edema is similar to highaltitude pulmonary edema, dexamethasone or acetazolamide may be useful.

Conclusion

Hormonal changes as a result of acute autonomic nervous system imbalance are frequent and typical in intracerebral hemorrhage, SAH, and ischemic stroke. There is a uniform pattern, with increases in norepinephrine, normetanephrine, and the reninangiotensinaldosterone system. Different mechanisms such as vasospasms, ICP rise, or hydrocephalus may cause these similar autonomic changes. Finally, there is a close prognostic relationship between hormonal excesses and bad outcomes.

Several unresolved questions remain: Is there a specific role for the autonomic dysbalance in generating ICP rises? Do hormonal changes play an additional role in generation of vasospasm? Can new imaging techniques clarify the relationship between location of the damage and the severity of autonomic changes? And finally, is the autonomic imbalance a result or a cause of the various complications seen in acute cerebrovascular disorder?

References

1. Cushing H. (1902) Some experimental and clinical observations concerning states of increased intracranial tension. The Mutter Lecture for 1901. American Journal of the Medial Sciences, September, 1902
2. Graf CJ, Rossi NP (1976) Catecholamine response to intracranial hypertension. J Neurosurg 49:862
3. Hamann G (1993) Autonome Veränderungen von lebensbedrohlichen intrakraniellen Erkrankungen. Habilitationsschrift, Hamburg, Saar
4. Hamann G, Haass A, Schimrick K (1993) Beta blockade in acute aneurysmal subarachnoid hemorrhage. Acta Neurochir 121:179
5. Simmons RL, Martin AM Jr, Heisterkamp CA, et al (1969) Respiratory insufficiency in combat casualties. II. Pulmonary edema following head injury. Ann Surg 170:139
6. Matjasko MJ (1994) Multisystem sequelae of severe head injury. In: Cottrell JE, Smith DS (eds) Anesthesia and Neurosurgery. Mosby, St. Louis, Missouri, pp 685
7. Malik AB (1977) Pulmonary vascular response to increase in intracranial pressure: role of sympathetic mechanisms. J Appl Physiol 42:335
8. Simon RP, Bayne LL, Naughton MP (1982) Left atrial pressure elevation recreates the altered lung lymph flow of seizures. J Appl Physiol 53:432
9. McClellan MD, Dauber IM, Weil JV (1989) Elevated intracranial pressure increases pulmonary vascular permeability to protein. J Appl Physiol 67:1185
10. Touho H, Karasawa J, Shishido H, et al (1989) Neurogenic pulmonary edema in the acute stage of hemorrhagic cerebrovascular disease. Neurosurg 25:762

Intracranial Pressure and Circulatory Management

A. Unterberg and M. Fink

Introduction

Intracranial pressure, cerebral perfusion pressure, and circulatory management play major roles in effective therapy of acute brain trauma and in emergency treatment of acute stroke. The key elements are to maintain cerebral perfusion pressure (CPP) above 70 mmHg and to use hemodynamic therapy including intravascular volume expansion to maintain cerebral perfusion and oxygen delivery to areas of ischemic tissue, with the goal of preventing reversible ischemia from progressing to irreversible infarction.

Intracranial Pressure Following Severe Head Injury

A. Unterberg

Key parameters guiding treatment of severely head-injured patients have changed considerably in the last 25 years. First neurological status examinations guided by simple scales were used. Then intracranial pressure (ICP) monitoring was introduced. Recently the importance of cerebral perfusion pressure (CPP) has been appreciated again [1]. However, CPP is important only to guarantee sufficient cerebral blood flow and cerebral oxygenation. Since routine monitoring of cerebral blood flow is not feasible, cerebral oxygenation monitoring has attracted more interest.

Guidelines

Generally accepted medical treatment of elevated ICP was codified in 1995 in the "Guidelines for the Management of Severe Head Injury" issued by the Joint Section on Neurotrauma and Critical Care of the American Association of Neurological Surgeons and the Congress of Neurological Surgeons [2]. Treatment approaches are presented as standards, guidelines, and options.

Standards represent an accepted principle of patient management that reflects a high degree of clinical certainty and is based on class 1 evidence: prospective randomized clinical trials. Guidelines represent a moderate level of clinical certainty and are based on retrospective analyses of prospectively collected data, observational studies, cohort studies, prevalence studies, or case-control studies.

Options are patient management strategies for which there is unclear clinical certainty and are based on retrospectively collected data, clinical series, case reviews, case reports, and expert opinion. ICP treatment should be initiated at an upper threshold of 20 to 25 mmHg.

The gold standard for monitoring ICP is a ventricular catheter plus external strain gauge. It is most accurate, low costs, reliable, can be recalibrated, and permits therapeutic CSF drainage. A second choice is parenchymal ICP monitoring. This is similar to the ventricular catheter but has a potential of drift and does not permit therapeutic drainage. Fluid-coupled epidural or subdural monitors and pneumatic epidural monitors are truly less accurate and therefore only a third choice.

Basic ICP Treatment

The guidelines for management of ICP in severe head injury say that treatment should be initiated at an upper threshold of 20–25 mmHg. The guideline for cerebral perfusion pressure, which is at the level of an option, says that CPP should be maintained at a minimum of 70 mmHg but may be elevated beyond this in individual circumstances.

The first step in the pathway for managing ICP is ventricular drainage of CSF, if possible. The second step is to introduce mannitol. Mannitol is effective for control of raised ICP after severe head injury. Limited data suggest that intermittent boluses may be more effective than continuous infusion. Effective doses range from 0.25 g/g body weight to 1 g/kg body weight. The third step is to start moderate hyperventilation ($PaCO_2$ 30–35 mmHg). The guidelines state as a standard that the use of prophylactic hyperventilation therapy should be avoided because it can compromise cerebral perfusion during a time when cerebral blood flow is reduced [3].

More recently use of hyperventilation has been discouraged, since hyperventilation impairs cerebral oxygenation [4]. As an option, hyperventilation therapy may be necessary for brief periods when there is acute neurologic deterioration or for longer periods if there is intracranial hypertension that is refractory to sedation, paralysis, CSF drainage, and osmotic diuretics.

Additional methods should be used to monitor this mode of treatment such as measurement of the arteriovenous difference of oxygen and/or cerebral blood flow monitoring. If these methods fail to reduce ICP below 20 mmHg, second-tier therapies for refractory intracranial hypertension are called for. These therapies are not proven to ameliorate outcome. They include barbiturates, surgical decompression, and hypertensive therapy. High-dose barbiturate therapy should be considered in hemodynamically stable severe head injury patients with intracranial hypertension refractory to maximal medical and surgical ICP lowering therapy.

Monitoring

Multimodal cerebral monitoring is a technique for improving the care of patients after traumatic brain injury. Optimal treatment of increased ICP requires monitoring not only ICP but also mean arterial blood pressure, perfusion pressure, end tidal CO2, arterial oxygenation, temperature, and perhaps oxygenation. Ideally, these data should be collected simultaneously.

We developed a system to sample, store, and analyze these data (Fig. 1). The hardware required includes an IBM-compatible personal computer with a Pentium chip, 32 MB of RAM, and a 1 GByte hard drive, and A/D converter board with 16 bits and 16 channels, a 32-channel multiplexer board, a MO disk with 1.3 MB and tape streamer, color monitor, termination board, laser printer, and uninterruptible power supply. Software includes Windows 95, LabVIEW 3.1.1 for Windows 95, SigmaPlot 3.0 for Windows 95, Word 7.0 for Windows 95, and LabVIEW-based multimodal cerebral monitoring (MCM) software.

Recently this system has been used to investigate severely (GCS < 8) head injured patients [5]. They were mostly younger patients (average age 24.6 years, range 15–66 years). The first question asked concerned the effect of changes in head position. Standard treatment is to elevate the head to 30 degrees. What happens if you lower the head to 0 degrees for 20 minutes? This was studied in 18 patients and 22 maneuvers. MCM revealed an increase in mean arterial blood pressure and an increase in ICP from 16 to about 24 mm Hg, which has been regarded as harmful. However, cerebral perfusion pressure increased slightly, and along with this cerebral oxygenation (measured by brain tissue pO_2 monitoring and jugular-venous oximetry) increased. The conclusion is that elevating the

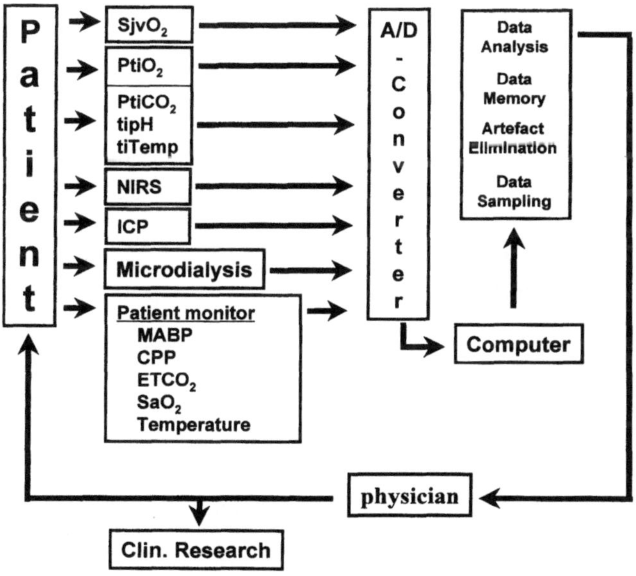

Fig. 1. Multimodal Cerebral Monitoring System

head to 30 degrees is not necessarily the optimal way to treat these patients (Fig. 2).

Cerebral perfusion pressure elevation was studied using a stepwise dopamine-induced increase of mean arterial blood pressure in 18 patients. Dopamine was given to a maximum dosage of 1.5 mg/min. In patients with initial spontaneous drop in arterial BP and with an initial CPP of below 50 mmHg, CPP climbed above 60 mm Hg after dopamine administration. This effectively increased both brain tissue pO_2 and jugular-venous oxygen saturation.

Thus, it is important to elevate the CPP above 60 mmHg at least. In patients with initial CPP greater than 60 mm Hg there was an additional CPP rise following the increase of mean arterial BP, but there was no significant additional rise in cerebral oxygenation. Mannitol (20%, 0.4 g/kg for 30 min) was administered if ICP was above 20, plasma osmolality was less than 320 mosmol/L, and renal function was normal. Mannitol was given to 5 patients during 16 maneuvers. ICP was effectively reduced by mannitol, CPP increased steadily, but the oxygenation of the brain did not improve significantly. This was apparently because the CPP was always above 60 mmHg in these patients. In such cases, although ICP was elevated, administration of mannitol is truly not necessary.

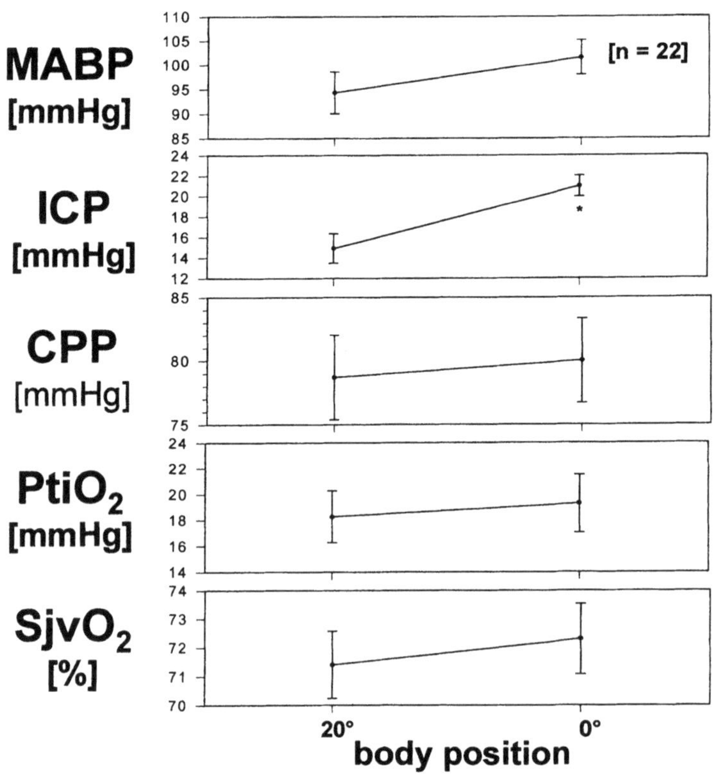

Fig. 2. Effect of Lowering Head Elevation to 0 Degrees

Hyperventilation was studied in 9 patients during 13 maneuvers. $ETCO_2$ was lowered by raising the respiratory rate for 10 minutes. The maneuver was terminated if oxygen saturation in the jugular vein ($SjvO_2$) decreased to less than 50 percent. This effectively reduced ICP and improved CPP, but it decreased oxygenation and may be harmful in cases where oxygenation is critical.

Summary of ICP Management

In summary, studies with multimodal cerebral monitoring have demonstrated the following about treatment of severely head-injured patients:
- Lowering the head to 0 degrees elevation had no influence on cerebral oxygenation
- Increasing CPP above 60 mmHg significantly improves cerebral oxygenation, but there is no benefit from further CPP elevation
- Mannitol infusion produced in improvement in cerebral oxygenation as long as CPP was above 60 mmHg
- Hyperventilation caused a significant worsening of cerebral oxygenation despite ICP reduction and CPP elevation
- Maintaining CPP above 70 mmHg will result in correct treatment in the majority of cases of severe head injury.

Therapy guided by CPP monitoring represents the current standard of care and preserves sufficient cerebral oxygenation in most cases.

Induced Hypertension in the Treatment of Acute Ischemic Stroke

M. Fink

There are three major goals in emergency treatment of acute ischemic stroke. The first is rapid recognition and treatment of focal ischemia. The second is neuronal protection. The third is restoration of blood flow to ischemic regions. There is unlikely to be a "magic bullet" that will suddenly and miraculously cure these patients, partly because the ability to apply specific treatment so often occurs only after the time period when there would be a possibility of success.

Hemodynamic therapy has been proven successful over the last 10–15 years in reducing the ischemic complications of aneurysmal subarachnoid hemorrhage in patients who present with focal brain ischemia [6, 7]. This approach can be applied to many patients in addition to other specific therapy and can be initiated immediately during transport or in the emergency department. Hemodynamic therapy has not yet been tested in randomized clinical trials, but it does conform with what is known about the relation of cerebral blood flow (CBF) to increased perfusion to areas of focal ischemia.

Hemodynamic therapy approaches must consider cardiovascular hemodynamics, cerebrovascular dynamics, and the impact of cardiovascular manipulations on CBF. Regulation of CBF in a healthy individual is determined by the cerebral metabolic rate for oxygen, arterial oxygen content, arterial carbon dioxide content, autoregulation, neurohumoral factors, and the hemorrheologic properties of blood (blood viscosity) [8, 9]. The two areas most accessible for therapeutic manipulation are blood pressure and blood viscosity.

Cerebral perfusion pressure is the difference between the mean arterial pressure and the intracranial pressure. Becker et al. showed in dogs the important relationship between arterial blood pressure and elevated ICP, specifically the pathogenesis of plateau waves (Fig. 3). The sudden rise ICP that occurs with a plateau wave is preceded by a small drop in systemic arterial pressure, which causes an even larger drop in cerebral perfusion pressure. This is followed by a massive, generalized vasodilatation of cerebral arterioles and a rise in ICP [10].

This has been translated into therapies including intentional elevation of CPP in patients with traumatic brain injury to reduce ICP and help prevent the development of fatal plateau waves. In the normal brain (Fig. 4) cerebral blood flow is relatively constant over a broad range of mean arterial blood pressures, from about 50 to about 150 mm Hg [1]. This is due to a direct myogenic response to wall tension but can be influenced by various factors including metabolic changes. Chronic hypertension shifts this curve to the right. Certain drugs, most typically the angiotensin-converting enzyme (ACE) inhibitors, shift the curve to the left. Ischemia or trauma can alter the response of the cerebral arteries so that the curve becomes a linear relationship between cerebral blood flow and arterial blood pressure.

Naritomi et al. studied changes in CBF in patients with vertebrobasilar ischemia due to transient ischemic attacks [11]. In this group of patients there was a loss of autoregulation in the posterior circulation so that CBF became a linear function of mean arterial blood pressure.

Animal studies have shown that arterial blood pressure is an important variable influencing outcome after ischemia [12, 13]. Other factors include duration of ischemia, degree of collaterals, the animal species used, pO_2, hematocrit, glucose, and core temperature [14].

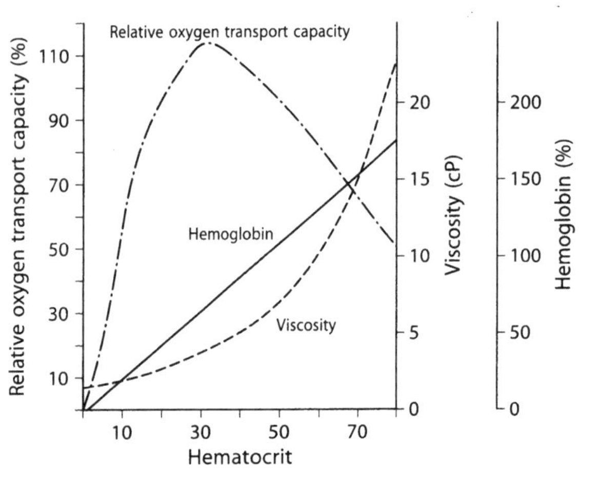

Fig. 3. Relationship between Systemic Arterial Pressure, Cerebral Perfusion Pressure, and Intracranial Pressure

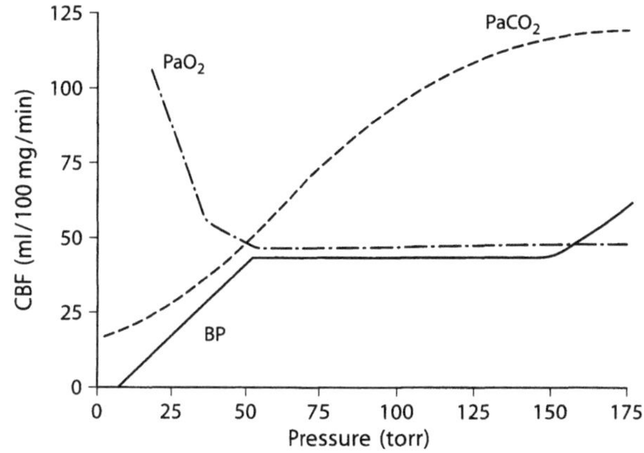

Fig. 4. Blood Pressure, PaO_2, $PaCO_2$, and Cerebral Blood Flow in the Normal Brain

Raising arterial blood pressure to improve cerebral perfusion is seldom an issue because most patients who come acutely to the hospital with brain infarcts or brain hemorrhages already have elevated blood pressure [15]. Such patients tend to have modest elevations of blood pressure for several days following the acute event, regardless of whether they had previous hypertension. Patients with chronic hypertension "reset" their level of autoregulation, so that the lower limit for cerebral ischemia is higher than for nonhypertensive patients.

Autoregulation may be lost in regions affected by ischemia or hemorrhage, but that loss is unpredictable and variable. Increased ICP may cause a fall in CBF or cerebral perfusion pressure. Post-stroke arterial hypertension is often the result of brain stem ischemia. Hypertension associated with stroke is often associated with high sympathetic activity and extraordinarily high levels of catecholamines in the blood. In aneurysmal subarachnoid hemorrhage, for example, the level of circulating catecholamines may reach those seen in patients with active pheochromocytomas [16].

Hypertensive Treatment

In general, the blood pressure should therefore be left alone in patients who present with acute focal brain ischemia and elevated blood pressure. Lowering the blood pressure is likely to exacerbate the ischemia. Artificially elevating the blood pressure may be indicated in the patient with progressing or intermittent neurological symptoms in the acute setting of focal brain ischemia and without typically elevated blood pressure [17]. However, some clinicians feel that this is best approached with hypervolemic, hypertensive hemodilution rather than with pressors. Prospective data demonstrating efficacy does not exist for either blood pressure elevation or hypervolemic hypertensive hemodilution therapy.

Physiologically, blood pressure and blood viscosity can be manipulated to improve cerebral blood flow. Reduction of blood viscosity will have a profound effect on blood flow to the microcirculation and to the tissues. Lowering the hematocrit from 45 to 35 will dramatically increase cerebral blood flow [9].

In conjunction with elevated blood pressure, this will improve perfusion in the areas of ischemic brain. and limit the progression of ischemic tissue to infarcted tissue. Hemodilution alone has not been effective as a treatment in 3 separate groups of stroke patients [18–20]. This may well be because oxygen delivery is constant over a range of different hematocrits (Fig. 5) [14].

We believe that intravascular volume expansion with concomitant blood pressure elevation is the first line of treatment in patients with acute focal brain ischemia. Volume expansion increases cardiac output and mean arterial blood pressure while decreasing blood viscosity. This increases regional cerebral blood flow in ischemia areas where autoregulation is lost. This is a standard approach in aneurysmal SAH [6, 7] but we find it is also effective in acute focal brain infarction when dealing with large vessel occlusive disease where there are likely to be intact collaterals, including occlusion of the internal carotid, middle cerebral, or basilar artery. Patients with lacunar syndromes or small-end arterial occlusions would not be expected to respond to this type of treatment since they are likely to have few collaterals. We have used this approach in patients with a crescendo pattern of transient ischemic attacks who were not responding to other therapies while awaiting surgery.

If volume expansion alone is not effective, the appropriate agent must be used to increase cardiac output and raise blood pressure. Anesthesiologists often use phenylephrine, a pure alpha agent which only s blood pressure and theoretically should have no local effect on cerebral blood vessels or intracranial pressure. However, since the objective is to increase both blood pressure and cardiac output, dopamine or dopamine and phenylephrine in combination is a more appropriate choice.

The goals are to maintain optimal blood flow in the setting of acute brain ischemia or increased ICP. Therapy must be individualized based on a number of

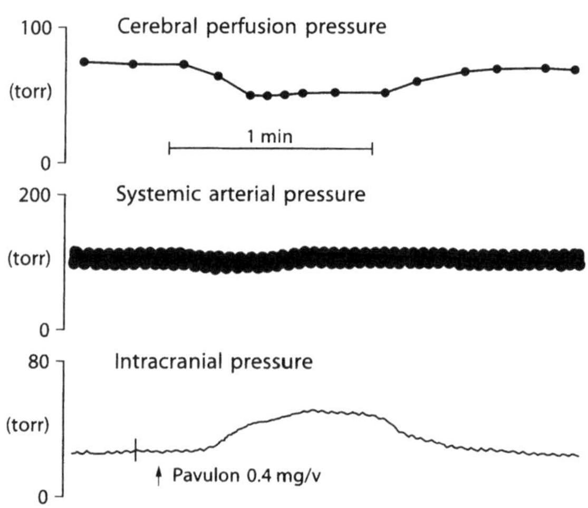

Fig. 5. Effect of Hematocrit on Oxygen Transport Capacity

important factors: presence or absence of pre-existing hypertension, location of the ischemic area, presence of intracranial hypertension, and status of the cardiopulmonary system. A reasonable therapeutic goal is to aim for incremental increase in the level of blood pressure below the upper level of autoregulation that will maximize CBF without exacerbating brain edema.

Conclusion

Management of ICP and closer attention to hemodynamic factors are emerging as important components in the optimal care of acute stroke. Multimodal, cerebral monitoring is extremely useful and has shown that maintaining CPP above 60 mmHg will correctly direct treatment in the majority of cases. Steps to lower ICP and protect cerebral perfusion should be initiated at an upper ICP threshold of 20–25 mmHg.

Blood pressure and blood viscosity are the two hemodynamic factors with greatest effect in focal brain ischemia. In general, blood pressure should not be lowered in patients with acute focal brain ischemia. Elevating blood pressure may be called for in patients who continue to deteriorate. Neurologically, this should ideally be done with hypervolemic hypertensive hemodilution rather than with pressors. If volume expansion alone is not sufficient, dopamine or dopamine and phenylephrine to augment cardiac output and blood pressure in an attempt to increase cerebral blood flow is indicated.

References

1. Rosner MJ, Rosner SD and Johnson AH (1995) Cerebral perfusion pressure: management protocol and clinical results. J Neurosurg 83:949–962
2. Bullock R, Ehsaman RM, Clifton G, et al (1996) Guidelines for the management of severe head injury. Brain Trauma Foundation. Eur J Emerg Med 3:109–127
3. Bouma GJ, Muizelaar JP, Choi SC, et al (1991) Cerebral circulation and metabolism after severe traumatic brain injury: the elusive role of ischemia. J Neurosurg 75:685–693
4. Dings J, Meixensberger J, Amschler J, et al (1966) Continuous monitoring of brain tissue PO2: a new tool to minimize the risk of ischemia caused by hyperventilation therapy. Zentralb Neurochir 57:177–183
5. Kiening KL, Unterberg AW, Bardt TF, et al (1996) Monitoring of cerebral oxygenation in patients with severe head injuries: brain tissue PO2 versus jugular vein oxygen saturation. J Neurosurg 85:751–757
6. Kassell NF, Peerless SJ, Durward QJ, et al (1982) Treatment of ischemic deficits from vasospasm with intravascular volume expansion and induced arterial hypertension. Neurosurgery 11:337–343
7. Haley EC Jr, Kassell NF, Torner JC (1993) A randomized controlled trial of high-dose intravenous nicardipine in aneurysmal subarachnoid hemorrhage. A report of the Cooperative Aneurysm Study. J Neurosurgery 78:537–547
8. Wagner EM, Traystman RJ (1985) Cerebrovascular transmural pressure and autoregulation. Annals of Biomedical Engineering 13:311–320
9. Waschke KF, Krieter H, Hagen G, et al (1994) Lack of dependence of cerebral blood flow on blood viscosity after blood exchange with a Newtonian O2 carrier. J Cerebral Blood Flow Metab 14:871–876

10. Rosner MJ and Becker DP (1984) Origin and evolution of plateau waves. Experimental observations and a theoretical model. J Neurosurgery 60:312–324
11. Naritomi H, Sakai F, Meyer JS (1979) Pathogenesis of transient ischemic attacks within the vertebrobasilar arterial system. Arch Neurol 36:121–128
12. Hayashi S, Nehls D, Kieck C, et al (1984) Beneficial effects of induced hypertension on experimental stroke in awake monkeys. J Neurosurgery 60:151–157
13. Cole D, Matsumura J, Drummond J, et al (1992) Focal cerebral ischemia in rats: effects of induced hypertension during reperfusion of CBF. J Cerebral Blood Flow Metab 12:64–69
14. Massik J, Tang YL, Hudak ML, et al (1987) Effect of hematocrit on cerebral blood flow with induced polycytemia. J Appl Physiol 62:1090–1096
15. Broderick J, Brott T, Barsan W, et al (1993) Blood pressure during the first minutes of focal cerebral ischemia. Annals of Emergency Medicine 22:1438–1443
16. Rivera Nava C, Corona T, Estanol B, et al (1994) Elevation of total urinary catecholamines in patients with subarachnoid hemorrhage. Rev Invest Clin 46:241–244
17. Rordorf G, Cramer S, Efird J, et al (1997) Pharmacological elevation of blood pressure in acute stroke. Clinical effects and safety. Stroke 28:2133–2138
18. Scandinavian Stroke Study Group (1987) Multicenter trial of hemodilution in acute ischemic stroke. Results in the total patient population. Stroke 18:291–299
19. Italian Acute Stroke Study Group (1988) Haemodilution in acute stroke: results of the Italian Haemodilution Trial. Lancet:318–326
20. The Hemodilution in Stroke Study Group (1989) Hypervolemic hemodilution treatment of acute stroke. Results of a randomized multicenter trial using pentastarch. Stroke 20:317–323

Imaging and the Early Evaluation of Stroke

E. B. Ringelstein, R. von Kummer, and J.-C. Baron

New imaging techniques are increasingly improving clinical decision-making in acute ischemic stroke. Computed Tomography (CT) and Positron Emission Tomography (PET) scans provide new ways to differentiate salvageable tissue from irreversible damage. Extracranial Doppler ultrasound, including color-coded B-mode imaging and transcranial Doppler sonography (TCD) can speed initial diagnostic work-up thus indirectly decreasing the risk of fibrinolysis [1–3]. PET has further altered previous thinking on the "therapeutic window" after acute ischemic stroke. As will be explained in more detail below, ultrasound can particularly speed up initial triage and diagnostic work-up of the acute stroke patient by demonstrating embolically active, high-grade stenoses or occlusions of the neck arteries (corresponding to the stroke), or embolic occlusions of the major brain arteries, particularly the MCA. TCD can also contribute to a more favorable outcome by proving that the occluding clot in the large pial arteries has already been lysed spontaneously making fibrinolysis superfluous. This is a very important role of TCD, to contribute to a more favorable outcome in these patients and to help reduce (or avoid) the complications of fibrinolysis.

Computed Tomography in Acute Ischemic Stroke: the Importance of Early Infarct Signs

Early signs of ischemic brain infarction on computed tomography (CT) are changes in x-ray attenuation which reflect thromboembolic arterial obstruction, ischemic brain edema, or brain tissue swelling and which can be recognized on the initial CT scan within the first few hours of stroke onset. We will discuss here how reliably these radiological phenomena can be assessed, what they are in terms of pathophysiology, and whether these findings are significant for the patient's prognosis and management.

The Hyperdense Artery Sign

The hyperdense artery sign is defined as hyperattenuation of a larger brain vessel, typically of the middle, posterior, anterior cerebral artery (MCA, PCA, ACA), or the distal internal carotid artery (ICA). "Hyperattenuation" means that a por-

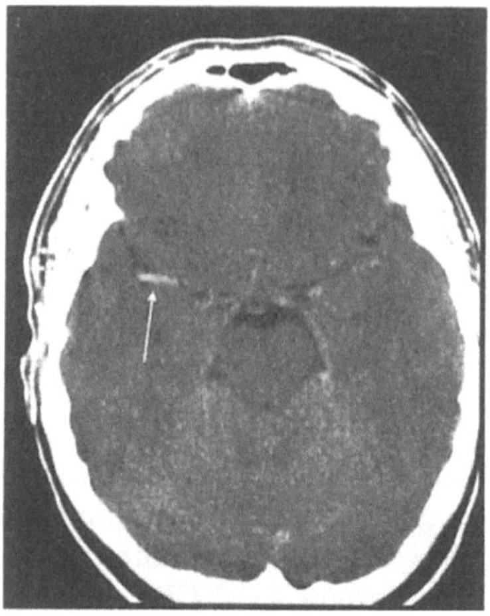

Fig. 1. Tubular shaped hyperattenuation in the right anterior sylvian fissure (arrow): the *h*yperdense *m*iddle cerebral *a*rtery *s*ign (HMCAS). The contralateral middle cerebral artery (MCA) appears slightly denser than brain parenchyma, but is not as dense as the right MCA trunk. This finding is highly specific for MCA trunk occlusion

tion of the artery is lighter on the scan than other portions of the same artery or of the contralateral artery (Fig. 1) [4]. The specificity of the hyperdense MCA sign (HMCAS) is 98% [5]. The sign is false positive in the case of unilateral calcification of the MCA trunk. The sensitivity of the HMCAS is quite low at about 50% [5]. The volume and composition of the thrombus may be responsible for the frequent false negative findings. The chance adjusted agreement among blinded readers is k=0.6 [6]. Disagreement can be explained by the different degrees of attenuation which are accepted as hyperattenuation by different readers of the CT scan.

The hyperdense artery sign proves that a major cerebral vessel is occluded and that this vessel's territory is at risk from hypoperfusion. Internal carotid artery and MCA trunk occlusions have more serious clinical implications than occlusions of MCA branches, the PCA, or the ACA because the resulting ischemic edema may be larger, and life threatening brain swelling can occur. The question to which extent the affected territory will undergo ischemic necrosis is a matter of collateral blood supply. Extremely different situations have been observed: The hyperdense artery sign can be associated with an immediate large ischemic edema covering the entire arterial territory or with a normal CT scan of brain tissue.

In case of the HMCAS, the infarction is often and typically restricted to the basal ganglia which have almost no collaterals in contrast to the brain cortex [7]. That means that this sign is literally not an *infarct* sign. It provides angiographic information and indicates the potential risk of infarction. It cannot predict the exact size of infarction, but indicates the volume of tissue which will die if the collateral blood supply fails and recanalization is not achieved. Clinically, the HMCAS is associated with a poor prognosis [4]. It is thus important to recognize the hyperdense artery sign. Moreover, it helps to better detect areas of subtle hypoattenuation because it defines the territory where ischemic edema may occur.

Focal Hypoattenuation

Electron density determines x-ray attenuation. When the brain tissue takes up water, x-ray attenuation is reduced by 2 to 3 Hounsfield units (HU) per 1% increase in tissue water concentration [8]. In brain areas with low perfusion (< 15 ml/100 g/min) – which is below the threshold of structural integrity – tissue water concentration increases by ~0.6% per hour immediately after arterial occlusion [9]. This water uptake is detected by CT which shows a linear decline in x-ray attenuation by ~1.5 HU per hour (J. Weber et al. unpublished data). Because of the normal noise in each image, a change of about 5 HU is necessary that an increase in tissue water becomes visible. That means that visible subtle hypoattenuation within the territory of an occluded artery means focal uptake of water of at least 2% and an arterial occlusion which occurred some time earlier (Fig. 2).

We presume that the time delay between arterial occlusion and visible hypoattenuation on CT scans is not only affected by the amount of water uptake – which may be determined by the degree of ischemia, but also by other factors influencing x-ray attenuation like the local cerebral blood volume (CBV). Focal vasodilation with an increase in CBV is a well known mechanism which compensates low perfusion pressure. In our series of 53 patients with proved MCA trunk occlusion, the earliest ischemic edema was visible at 46 minutes after stroke onset, and all CT scans obtained after 132 minutes after the onset of symptoms showed a hypoattenuated area [5]. We must, therefore, take into account that we may not detect large ongoing ischemic edema during the first two hours.

If the initial CT shows, however, hypoattenuated tissue, such CT findings mean identification of a volume of tissue which underwent severe ischemia and is irreversibly damaged. If this volume is large, focal brain swelling will considerably increase the intracranial pressure, decrease perfusion pressure and thus deter-

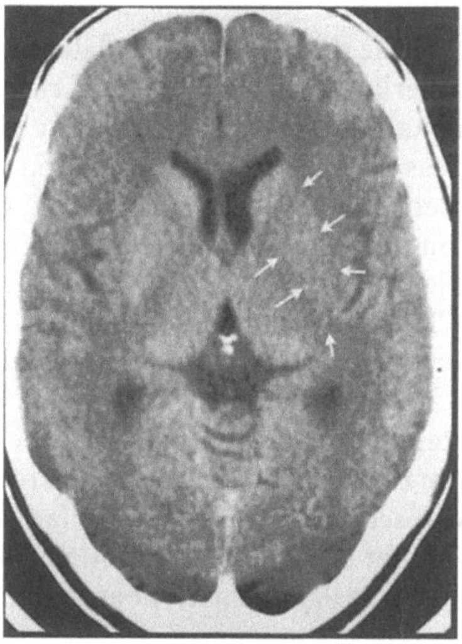

Fig. 2. The left lentiform nucleus (arrows) is still denser than the surrounding white matter tracks (internal and external capsule), but clearly less dense in comparison to the right lentiform nucleus. Its margins are already somewhat blurred. These findings mean early development of ischemic edema and subsequent necrosis

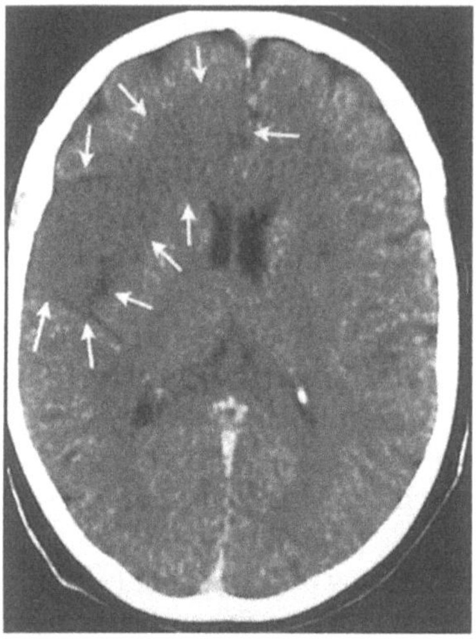

Fig. 3. Large early ischemic edema in the middle and anterior cerebral artery territories depicted by CT 3 hours after symptom onset. The hypoattenuation is already marked and exceeds one third of the MCA territory (at least in this section)

mine the clinical course (Fig. 3). We do not think that an ischemic edema – detected by CT with some delay – will benefit from arterial recanalization and reperfusion. Reperfusion may further enhance edema in areas of dense ischemia [10]. It makes no sense to apply thrombolytic agents to achieve recanalization, if the majority of an arterial territory already shows edema [11].

This consideration is the rationale for the decision not to include patients with an ischemic edema exceeding one third of the MCA territory into the European Cooperative Acute Stroke Study (ECASS) [12]. This study finally showed that patients – falsely randomized – with such large edema did not benefit from thrombolysis and had an increased risk for brain parenchymal hematomas if treated with intravenous recombinant tissue plasminogen activator (rt-PA, 1.1 mg/kg) [13].

These first prospective data on the CT findings prior to thrombolytic therapy underline the importance of carefully reading the initial CT scan of stroke patients. For an experienced, but blinded reader it may be possible to detect all areas of subtle hypoattenuation on early CT scans [16]. The chance adjusted interobserver agreement among 6 neuroradiologists was $k=0.58$ for the detection of hypoattenuation and $k=0.65$ for the estimate of the extent of such areas [6].

This moderate to good agreement reflects the fact that early ischemic edema is represented by a very subtle decrease in x-ray attenuation by less than 10 HU. It first appears on a CT scan by a loss of anatomical information [15, 16]. Hypoattenuation of the lentiform nucleus or the insular cortex makes these structure undiscernible from the surrounding white matter. Unfortunately, an oblique scan section can cause a similar phenomenon. The reader has to carefully check whether e.g. an "obscuration of the lentiform nucleus" or "loss of the insular ribbon" is really due to hypoattenuation and not to section obliquity.

Focal Brain Swelling

Brain swelling is very subtle during the first hours after arterial occlusion. Swelling of brain tissue is assessed on CT scans by looking for the compression of the cerebrospinal fluid (CSF) spaces and the focal enlargement of structures like the cortex (Fig. 4). Because of the natural asymmetry of the brain's sulci and ventricles, it is hard to reliably assess early stages of brain swelling by comparing the CSF spaces of the two hemispheres. The interobserver agreement for signs of swelling on early CT scans among the above mentioned 6 neuroradiologists was in a similar range as for hypoattenuation with a $k=0.59$ [6].

In the ECASS, the initial CT scans of 129 patients (21%) showed focal brain swelling. Brain swelling was not detected in 144 patients (54%) out of 267 patients with already visible ischemic edema. In 6 patients, the swelling was not accompanied by a visible ischemic edema (2% of all patients without any early signs of infarction). Three patients with swelling on their initial CT scan had a normal CT on day 1 and day 7 after stroke onset. On the other hand, CT signs of early brain swelling were associated with poor prognosis ($p<0.001$).

We presume that focal brain swelling after arterial occlusion is caused either by compensatory focal vasodilation or by the developing ischemic edema. The space occupying effect of the very early edema may too subtle to be detected by CT. If swelling is visible, however, within the first 6 hours of stroke onset, it indicates severe edema and means poor prognosis for the majority of patients. Brain swelling caused by vasodilation alone may have a better prognosis. It is known from cerebral venous obstruction that arterial vasodilation is a reversible phenomenon and does not mean tissue damage [17].

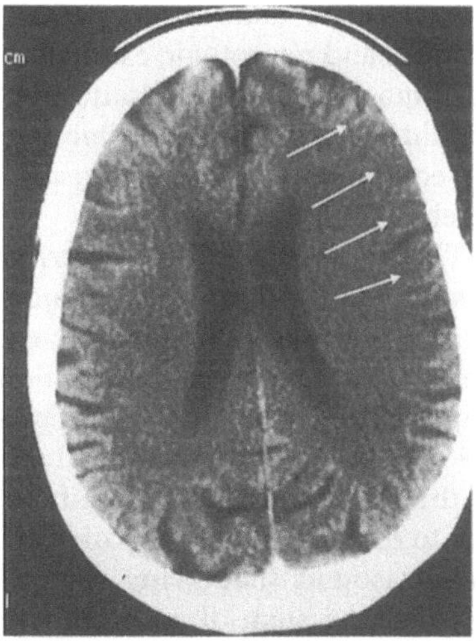

Fig. 4. Subtle focal effacement of cortical sulci in the left frontal lobe (arrows). If this finding is confirmed by other sections of this scan, focal brain swelling caused by edema or increase in local blood volume can be diagnosed

Transcranial Doppler Sonography

The emergency ultrasound approach depends on the stroke distribution. Stroke in the carotid distribution would typically require color-coded B-mode of the internal carotid artery (ICA), common carotid artery (CCA) and brachiocephalic trunk; transcranial Doppler ultrasound of the middle cerebral artery (MCA) carotid siphon, posterior cerebral artery (PCA) and anterior cerebral artery (ACA). TCD is also applied to the retromandibular (still extracranial) ICA to look for ICA dissections. In cases with lack of an ultrasound window in the temporal bone, echo contrast agents are used.

Stroke in the vertebrobasilar distribution would call for color-coded B-mode imaging of the extracranial vertebral arteries and the subclavian arteries as well, and for TCD of the distal vertebral arteries (including the intradural segment), the basilar artery, and the PCA. Again, echo contrast agents are used if there is lack of an adequate ultrasound window, or hypoplasia, or tortuosity of the vertebrobasilar vessels. Stroke of clinically equivocal distribution requires the evaluation of both the anterior and posterior circulation.

Once CT is done, ultrasound may be as reliable as arteriography for the majority of stroke-associated arterial lesions. This is, of course, only true if the laboratory involved is experienced. Ultrasound helps to prevent arteriography and may even be complementary to it [18, 19]. Ultrasonography will permit the use of fewer angiographies by allowing a more rapid and non-invasive evaluation of the cerebrovascular anatomy. Decisive advantage of ultrasound studies is that they can be repeated and are therefore ideal to guide aggressive treatment. If necessary, ultrasound is enhanced by use of echocontrast agents. In the future, it might be further improved by ultrasound based perfusion imaging. Ultrasound is expected to improve acute stroke care by permitting embolus detection to identify the active source of embolism in a very cost-effective manner. Presently, TCD is the only available technology at all to detect microembolism [20].

In triage of acute stroke patients, the first step is a quick history taking and a physical and neurologic exam of the patient. This should be followed by computed tomography of the brain and ultrasound screening of the vasculature. CT should be done first if possible, but TCD can be done first to save time in case that CT equipment is busy. The reason for the timely priority of CT is to check for cerebral hemorrhages.

The investigator should determine whether stroke is in the carotid or vertebrobasilar distribution. In the majority of cases, this can be evaluated by clinical means. If stroke symptoms are equivocal, however, physicians should first concentrate on the carotid distribution which has the highest probability of containing the stroke-causing lesion. The same holds true for the extracranial approach (as opposed to the intracranial tests). Color-coded B-mode imaging is the state-of-the-art technique to identify very high-grade or even subtotal ICA stenoses due to echolucent clots or calcified plaques even if the image is partially masked by ultrasound shadowing (Fig. 5). Color-coded B-mode ultrasound can even visualize the stem of an occluded ICA and permits a very reliable decision on whether the patient has total occlusion or "near occlusion" (so-called "pseudo-

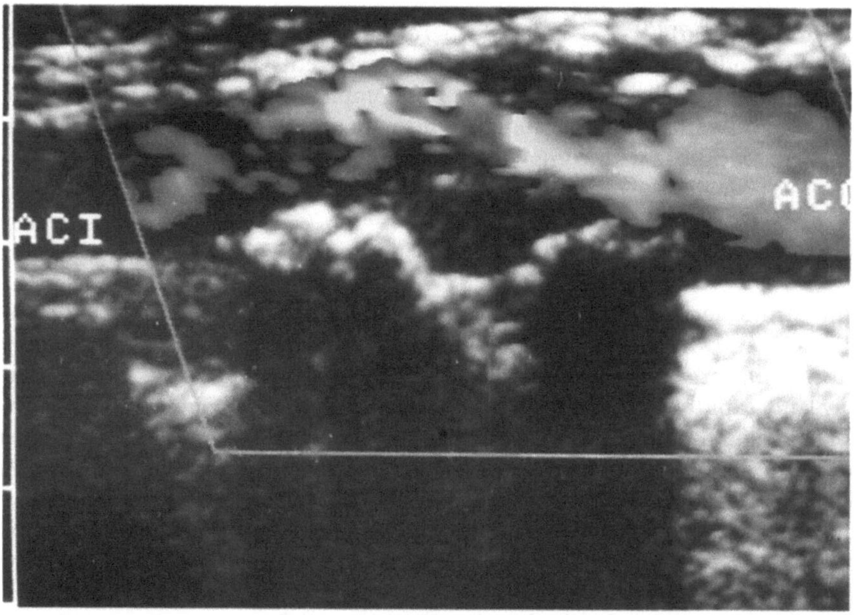

Fig. 5. High-grade ICA stenosis evaluated by color-coded B-mode imaging

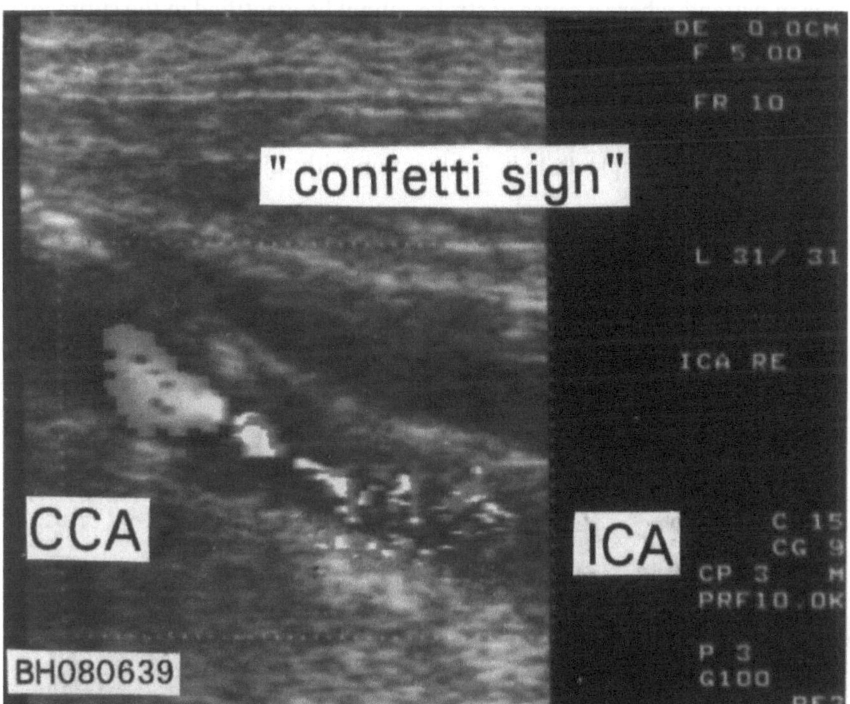

Fig. 6. Pseudoocclusion of the internal carotid artery

occlusion") (Fig. 6) [21–23]. In cases where a final decision cannot be made even with color-coding, the injection of echocontrast agents can lead to a final differentiation between pseudoocclusion versus complete occlusion. This differentiation is clinically important because patients with pseudoocclusion can be operated on, whereas those with complete occlusions cannot.

Specific TCD Approaches in Acute Stroke

In the carotid territory, the circle of Willis and its main feeding arteries (i.e. the distal ICA and the basilar artery) should be visualized, as well as their main branches, the large leptomeningeal arteries (MCA, PCA, ACA). This can be done easily and rapidly by means of transcranial color-coded Duplex sonography (TCCD) (Fig. 7). With the additional help of echocontrast agents, it is now even possible to make a relatively reliable diagnosis in the M_2-segment of the MCA. Occlusions at this site are relatively rare and hard to detect, but we can at least diagnose stenoses by very high-grade flow velocities at shallow insonation depths between 35 and 30 mm. TCCD makes it possible to visualize the cerebrovascular system by tracking the large arteries step by step and looking at the flow velocities and spectra to decide whether there is abnormal flow or not.

Transoesophageal echocardiography is also being used in stroke units for rapid triage in patients where a cause of stroke cannot be identified in the supraaortic vasculature. This is particularly important because of sources of embolism in the heart itself and in areas near the heart. "Pericardiac" sources of embolism, such as the aortic arch or intracardiac shunts, are not infrequent. Transoesophageal echocardiography can identify patients with patent foramen ovale, but this can also be done by simple TCD in conjunction with injection of echocontrast

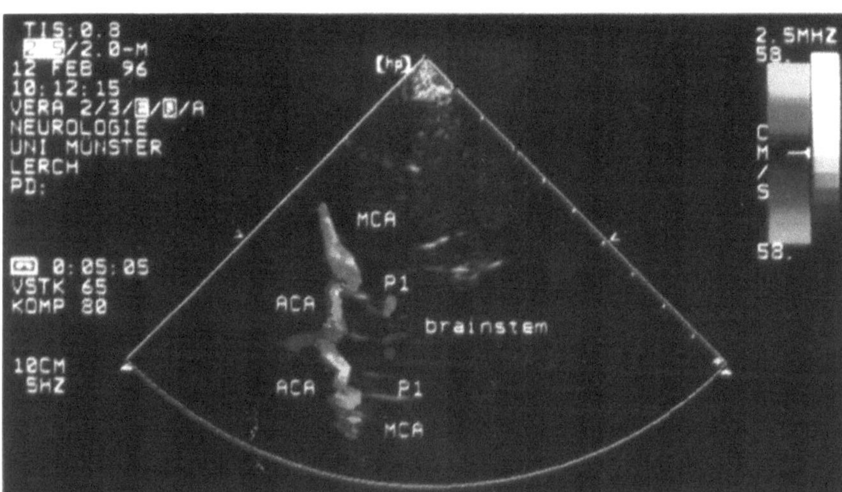

Fig. 7. Color-coded Duplex sonography of the circle of Willis

agents. If showers of gaseous emboli (not single bubbles) occur within a certain time frame within the cerebral arteries, they indicate the presence of an intracardiac shunt of critical size [24]. This technique helps to pinpoint the cause of stroke in so-called "cryptogenic" patients.

Microembolus Detection

This time consuming technique, though very promising, is still not suitable for the management of stroke patients in the very acute phase. Under certain circumstances, however, particularly with multiple potential sources of embolism, the bilateral 30–60 minutes monitoring of flow signals of the major pial arteries (e.g. the left and right MCA, or the MCA on one side and the PCA on the other side) may deliver decisive clues for the identification of the true, embolically active lesion and its delineation from innocent bystanders. Microemboli create a characteristic echo both visually on the screen and acoustically (Fig. 8). Microemboli are clinically silent, nevertheless they are indicators of an increased risk of further embolism and stroke [25, 26]. Repetitive screenings for the hourly rate of microemboli can be of decisive help to guide treatment, like dosage of antiplatelet agents, anticoagulants or combinations of them. A minimum of 30-minute recordings are necessary, 1-hour recordings are recommended [27].

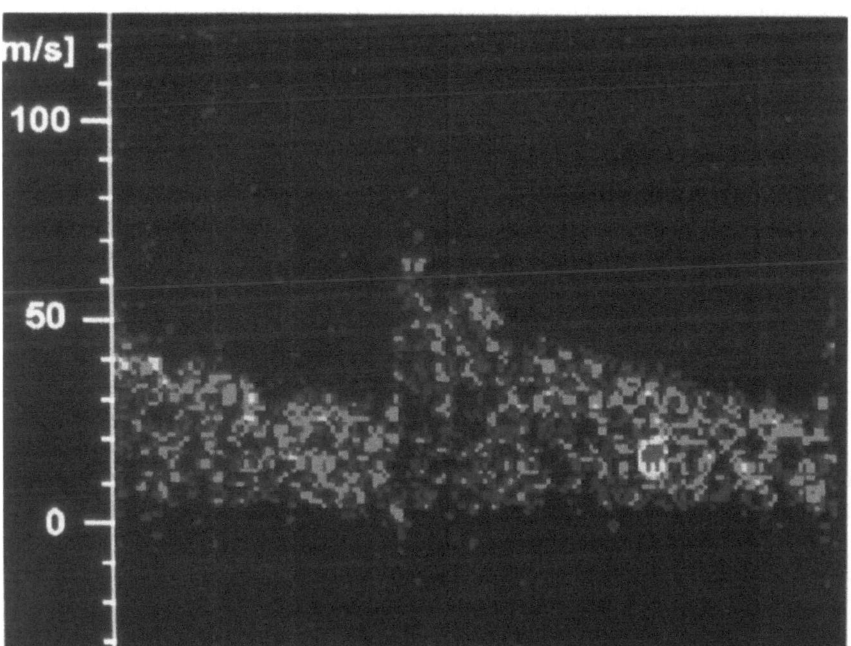

Fig. 8. Microembolus within the normal flow signal of the middle cerebral artery

Considerations with Leptomeningeal Anastomoses

The presence or absence of leptomeningeal anastomoses is an important prognostic factor in MCA occlusions. If these anastomoses are perfect, the patient usually has a small infarction only, either in the insular cortex or the basal ganglia ("striatocapsular infarction") [28]. The reduction of the size of the lesions is due to retrograde flow through the MCA branches fed by the leptomeningeal anastomoses from the anterior or posterior cerebral arteries. If this flow is only moderate, the patient is a candidate for thrombolytic therapy and for neuroprotection. If, however, there is no retrograde flow at all but a still complete occlusion of the MCA, the patient is probably not a candidate for fibrinolysis because the infarction is likely to be large, the risk of cerebral bleeding is increased and the outcome is likely to be poor. The presence of leptomeningeal anastomoses is difficult to assess by ultrasound. Abnormally high flow velocities in the main stems of the nonoccluded, ipsilateral PCA or ACA are an indirect indicator of major transcortical flow to the ischemic MCA territory. Arteriography is the method of choice. PET studies (see below) may also be helpful to evaluate the extent of collateral blood supply to the distribution the main feeding artery of which is still occluded. Perfusion Imaging techniques are expected to become the future tools to clarify this clinically important issue. Contrast enhanced color-flow imaging may also be helpful in defining the sufficiency of the leptomeningeal collaterals in that it means allow imaging of the very slow reflux within the main MCA branches distal to the proximal MCA occlusion. At the moment, CT-arteriography by spiral-computerized tomography seems to be the method of choice to visualize the MCA branches distal to a proximal occlusion; but these images do not provide any information about the flow direction, the flow velocity, or the volume of the reflux [29].

Use of Ultrasound with Fibrinolysis

Ultrasound can help in the primary and repetitive diagnosis of MCA occlusion by indicating whether the lesion is present at all, still present or already recanalized. TCD can also differentiate occlusion from subtotal stenosis. Perhaps the most important benefit is that ultrasound can confirm the clinical diagnosis, can be done repetitively and close to the anticipated time of fibrinolysis. This is particularly important because there are many cases of patients transported to the angiography suite lying already on the table ready for arteriography whose arteries had spontaneously reopened meanwhile by endogenous fibrinolysis. A confirmatory ultrasound investigation before arteriography is the key to prevent unnecessary exogenous fibrinolysis, which bears a high risk of intracranial bleeding [30]. In an observational study in 34 patients seen in the first 12 hours after stroke, we could assess spontaneous recanalization in the majority of them [1]. All patients had MCA occlusion on admission, detected either by angiography or by TCD. They were reinvestigated by TCD within very short time frames, namely at 2, 3, 4, 12, 20 and 44 hours poststroke. Further checks were performed on days 3, 10 and 17. Within 72 hours, occlusion had spontaneously opened in nearly two thirds of the patients (Fig. 9a). Similar findings have been seen by others as well [31, 32]. These findings underline how quickly a therapeutic (i.e. exogenous) fibrinolytic agent must be administered to have the chance to enhance the normal spontaneous (i.e. endogenous) recanalization process in embolic MCA occlusions.

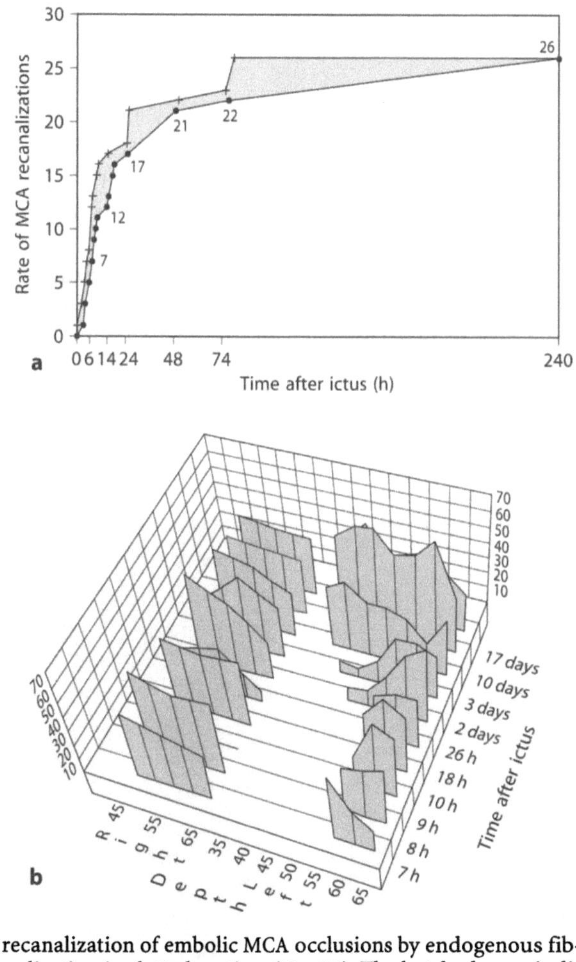

Fig. 9. a Diagram of spontaneous recanalization of embolic MCA occlusions by endogenous fibrinolysis. Frequency of MCA recanalization is plotted vs. time (N = 34). The hatched zone indicates the recanalization period, i.e. the time span within reopening of the MCA must have occurred. The majority of cases (21/34) had MCA recanalization within the first 48 hours (from Ringelstein et al. 1992). **b** Plot of TCD findings in an illustrative case with MCA recanalization. In leftsided MCA occlusion, an MCA flow signal was initially lacking at insonation depth of 45 and 50 mm. 26 hours and two days after the ictus, low flow velocities could be found within the proximal MCA, indicating partial recanalization. On day 3, hyperperfusion began to occur within the MCA and was most pronounced on day 10. Zero on time axis corresponds to time of onset of stroke

Another advantage of TCD is that it permits the immediate detection of bleeding within the cerebral parenchyma prompting interruption of rtPA treatment [33].

Reperfusion Injury and "No Reflow"

TCD also permits the determination of whether the patient has low flow reperfusion or hyperperfusion (Fig. 9b).

Titration of Fibrinolysis

Ultrasound can also help to tailor therapeutic "exogenous" fibrinolysis by means of recombinant tissue plasminogen activator (rtPA) [33]. For example, in patients with an MCA occlusion, the MCA stem may already reopen after 50 mg of rtPA instead of 100 mg usually to be infused. The ultrasound proof of recanalization permits stoppage of treatment, resulting in lower dosages of fibrinolytics and lower risk of bleeding (Fig. 10).

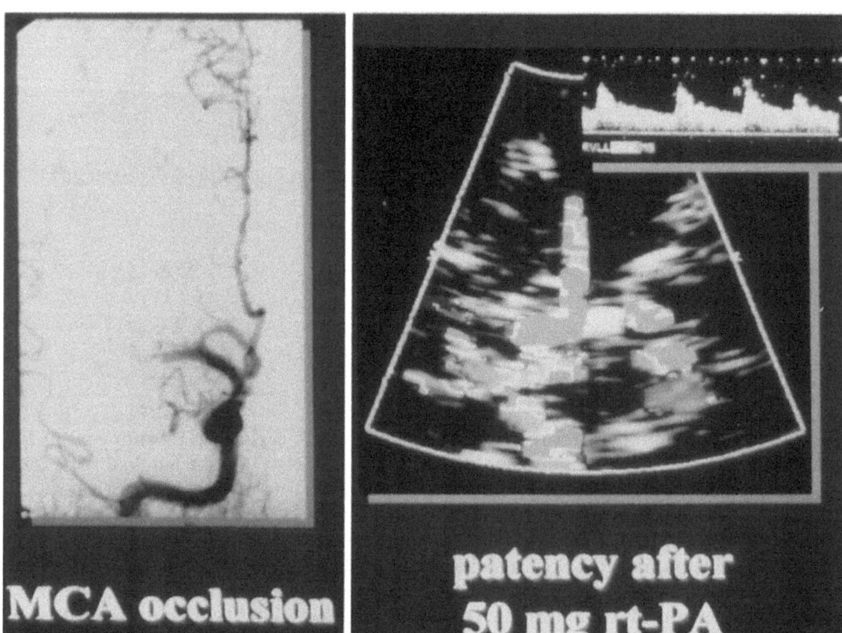

Fig. 10. Tailored fibrinolysis

PET Investigations in Acute Focal Cerebral Ischemia

The ischemic core in focal cerebral ischemia is the irreversibly damaged tissue in the central lesion. Around this is the ischemic penumbra, a rim of electrically disrupted neurons that are at risk but salvageable, provided appropriate measures are taken within the window of therapeutic opportunity. The volume of penumbral tissue shrinks, and little remains after a few hours in the awake monkey [34].

The ischemic penumbra is also characterized by reduced perfusion, with CBF typically <20 ml/100 g/min. There has been some debate over the benefit of rapidly restoring perfusion. However, spontaneous arterial recanalization occurs within six hours of stroke onset in about one-third of patients with MCA occlusion [35].

The penumbra can be documented by imaging both brain perfusion and regional oxygen consumption, which is an indication of cellular energy metabolism and basal synaptic activity. Determining how much penumbral tissue still exists in a given patient would allow us to select patients most likely to benefit from neuroprotective agents and to monitor the effects of such therapy.

Positron emission tomography (PET) is the only presently available technique that can produce quantitative maps of CBF, of the cerebral blood volume (CBV), and of the cerebral metabolic rate of oxygen ($CMRO_2$) [36]. PET also permits calculation of the CBV/CBF ratio, which represents the local circulatory mean transit time, and the CBF/CBV ratio, which reflects local cerebral perfusion pressure (CPP) [37, 38]. Quantitative maps of the oxygen extraction fraction (OEF) can be obtained using CBF and $CMRO_2$. Furthermore, all of these measurements can be obtained in a single 45-minute session and can be repeated over time.

Coupling and Uncoupling Among CBF, CBV, and $CMRO_2$

Under normal conditions, CBF, $CMRO_2$, and CBV vary according to linear relationships [20]. When CPP falls below the limits of autoregulation, the CBF also drops, but the $CMRO_2$ is sustained for some time. This "misery perfusion" results in a focal increase in the OEF up to the theoretical maximum of 1.00 and allows the brain to maintain its oxygen use despite reduced cerebral flow. Further drops in CPP, of course, cause true ischemia and impaired neuronal function [38]. There are thus two stages to ischemic damage: the penumbra, which is potentially reversible, and irreversible ischemia.

PET studies, in conjunction with CT scanning, have shown that salvageable tissue is distinguishable from necrotic areas by well-defined CBF and $CMRO_2$ threshold values [40]. Gray matter generally progress to infarction if it has $CMRO_2$ below 1.3–1.5 ml/100 g/min more than 2–6 hours after stroke [41, 42]. Tissue with values above this are sometimes salvageable, consistent with the concept of potentially reversible ischemia in the penumbra.

The hallmark of luxury perfusion (oxygen supply in excess of demand) is a focal reduction of the OEF seen on PET. This indicates that perfusion has been reestablished.

CBF and Metabolism in Acute Ischemic Stroke

Irreversibly damaged tissue, defined by profoundly reduced $CMRO_2$, affects the deep MCA territory very early and is often associated with misery perfusion [43, 44]. Marchal et al. [45] have shown that the volume of tissue with $CMRO_2$ below 1.5 ml/100 g/min as assessed with PET 5 to 18 hours post-onset of stroke is highly correlated with final infarct volume, as measured by CT scan one month later. Mapping the profoundly hypometabolic tissue in the acute stage of stroke may be helpful in predicting the minimum volume of the final infarction.

Early Hyperperfusion

In our sample of 10 patients with early hyperperfusion (which indicates recanalization of the occluded artery), the hyperperfused areas consistently maintained intact morphology over the longer term [46]. This suggests that early reperfusion after stroke in humans is a beneficial event.

Penumbral Tissue

One major discovery from PET studies is that ischemic but potentially reversibly damaged tissue is present even hours after the onset of stroke. The transition of such penumbral areas into infarction is characterized by a sharp decline in $CMRO_2$ despite CBF [47]. PET also reveals the progressive exhaustion of the tissue's oxygen as a dramatic fall in the OEF. Marchal et al. [48] recently used a sophisticated analysis of CT-coregistered PET data to map the part of the final infarct which was still potentially reversible 6–16 hours after stroke onset. This tissue still had oxygen consumption above 1.4 ml/100 g/min, and it represented 10 to 50% of the final infarct volume. This suggests that a substantial amount of ischemic damage is potentially reversible as late as 16 hours after clinical onset of acute stroke.

Marchal et al. also conducted the only systematic assessment of the relationship between acute-stage PET findings and clinical outcome [44,49]. They studied 30 patients with MCA territory stoke. Changes in CBF and $CMRO_2$ were studied 5–18 hours post-onset and compared to the neurological course over two months, quantitated with valid stroke scales. This revealed three patterns of PET changes.

Pattern 1 patients had large subcortico-cortical areas of extensive necrosis. Patter 2 patients had markedly reduced CBF but normal or relatively preserved $CMRO_2$, except in small and often deeply seated areas. This reflects ongoing ischemia with still limited necrosis. Pattern 3 patients had hyperperfusion with either essentially normal $CMRO_2$ or a limited area of profound hypometabolism. This reflects early spontaneous reperfusion and limited damage.

As might be expected, Patter 1 patients did poorly, Pattern 3 patients did well, and Pattern 2 patients had variable courses, ranging from death to full recovery.

These findings were the first to document the well-known clinical heterogeneity of stroke patients. It implies that since Pattern 1 and Pattern 3 patients are unlikely to benefit from therapy, including them in therapeutic trials may obscure any beneficial effect of the drug being tested. Pattern 2 patients may represent the subgroup most likely to benefit from therapeutic trials.

Furlan et al. [50] tested this hypothesis by attempting to correlate the outcomes of Pattern 2 patients to the outcome of the penumbra. They found that the volume of the ultimately non-infarcted penumbra strongly influenced subsequent neurological recovery.

There is one additional therapeutic implication of these PET findings. Patients with high OEF in the setting of acute stroke are having their autoregulation of CBF overridden in the affected territory. Lowering the systemic arterial pressure is likely to further reduce the cerebral perfusion pressure and CBF in the affected tissue, which may add to the damage in penumbral tissue. This may explain why reductions in systemic arterial pressure are associated with poorer outcomes in the setting of acute stroke [51].

On the other hand, patients with low OEF with hyperfusion may benefit from management of arterial hypertension, particularly if early edema is demonstrated by CT or MRI. Hyperperfusion in necrotic tissue may promote malignant brain swelling.

Future Hopes

The dream of sonographers at the moment is parenchymal monitoring by means of tissue perfusion. Unfortunately, this goal has not been reached yet. Further developments are likely to include color-coded imaging of retrogradely perfused MCA branches, more refined parenchymal imaging for hemorrhagic transformation and bleeding, and tissue perfusion imaging. Ultrasound is in general complementary to arteriography but may be superior in that it can be repeated ad libitum. Ultrasound techniques are ideal to guide aggressive types of treatment and reduce the associated risks. The validity of the ultrasound approach in diagnostically difficult situations has been enhanced considerably by the use of echocontract agents. Finally, important insights into acute stroke pathophysiology are likely to derive from ultrasound studies on embolus detection at multiple sites identifying and pinpointing the true source of embolism in ambiguous situations, e.g. multiple "competing" sources of embolism.

Conclusion

Computed tomography provides important information for patient management in acute stroke by assessing the affected arterial territory and the state and extent of ischemic edema. PET imaging suggests that the window of opportunity for neuroprotection is longer than had been predicted and may provide a tool for selecting potential responders to therapeutic intervention.

References

1. Ringelstein E, Biniek R, Weiller C, Ammeling B, Nolte P Thron A (1992) Type and extent of hemispheric brain infarctions and clinical outcome in early and delayed middle cerebral artery recanalization. Neurology 42:289–298
2. Karnik R, Stelzer, P, Slany J (1992) Transcranial Doppler sonography monitoring of local intra-arterial thrombolysis in acute occlusion of the middle cerebral artery. Stroke 23: 284–287
3. Seidel G, Kaps M, Gerriets T (1995) Potential and limitations of transcranial colour-coded sonography in stroke patients. Stroke 26:2061–2066
4. Tomsick T, Brott T, Barsan W (1992) Thrombus localization with emergency cerebral CT. AJNR Am J Neuroradiol 13:257–263
5. von Kummer R, Meyding-Lamadé U, Forsting M, et al (1994) Sensitivity and prognostic value of early computed tomography in middle cerebral artery trunk occlusion. AJNR Am J Neuroradiol 15:9–15
6. von Kummer R, Holle R, Grzyska U, et al (1996) Interobserver agreement in assessing early CT signs of middle cerebral artery infarction. AJNR Am J Neuroradiol 17:1743–1748
7. Bozzao L, Bastianello S, Fantozzi LM, et al (1989) Correlation of angiographic and sequential CT findings in patients with evolving cerebral infarction. AJNR Am J Neuroradiol 10: 1215–1222
8. Unger E, Littlefild J, Gado M (1988) Water content and water structure in CT and MR signal changes: Possible influence in detection of early stroke. AJNR Am J Neuroradiol 9: 687–691
9. Schuir FJ, Hossmann KA (1980) Experimental brain infarcts in cats. II. Ischemic brain edema. Stroke 11:593–601
10. Ianotti F, Hoff J (1983) Ischemic brain edema with and without reperfusion: An experimental study in gerbils. Stroke 14:562–567
11. von Kummer R, Holle R, Rosin L (1995) Does arterial recanalization improve outcome in carotid territory stroke? Stroke 26:581–587
12. Hacke W, Kaste M, Fieschi C, et al (1995) Safety and efficacy of intravenous thrombolysis with a recombinant tissue plasminogen activator in the treatment of acute hemispheric stroke. JAMA 274:1017–25
13. von Kummer R, Allen K, Holle R, et al (1997) Acute stroke: Usefulness of early CT findings before thrombolytic therapy. Radiology 205:327–333
14. von Kummer R, Nolte PN, Schnittger H (1996) Detectability of hemispheric ischemic infarction by computed tomography within 6 hours after stroke. Neuroradiology 38:31–33
15. Tomura N, Uemura K, Inugami A, (1988) Early CT finding in cerebral infarction. Radiology 168:463–467
16. Truwit CL, Barkovich AJ, Gean-Marton A, et al (1990) Loss of the insular ribbon: Another early CT sign of acute middle cerebral artery infarction. Radiology 176:801–806
17. Yuh W, Simonson T, Wang A, et al (1994) Venous sinus occlusive Disease: MR Findings. AJNR Am J Neuroradiol 15:309–316
18. Ley-Pozo J, Ringelstein E (1990) Noninvasive detection of occlusive disease of the carotid siphon and middle cerebral artery. Ann Neurol 28:640–647
19. Rorick MB, Nichols FT, Adams RJ (1994) Transcranial Doppler correlation with angiography in detection of intracranial stenoses. Stroke 25:1931–1934
20. Droste DW, Hansberg T, Kemény V, et al (1997) Oxygen inhalation can differentiate gaseous from non-gaseous microemboli detected by transcranial Doppler ultrasound. Stroke (in press)
21. Ringelstein EB, Berg-Dammer E, Zeumer H (1983) The so-called atheromatous pseudoocclusion of the internal carotid artery. Neuroradiology 25:147–155
22. Görtler M, Niethammer R, Widder B (1994) differentiating subtotal carotid artery stenoses from occlusions by colour-coded duplex sonography. J Neurol 241:301–305
23. Berman SS, Devine JJ, Erdoes LS, Hunter GC (1995) Distinguishing carotid artery pseudoocclusion with colour-flow Doppler. Stroke 26:434–438

24. Job FP, Ringelstein EB, Grafen Y, et al (1994) Comparison of transcranial Doppler sonography and transoesophageal contrast echocardiography in the detection of patent foramen ovale in young stroke patients. Am J Cardiol 74:381–384
25. Siebler M, Sitzer M, Rose G, Steinmetz H (1995) Cerebral microembolism and the risk of ischemia in asymptomatic high-grade internal carotid artery stenosis. Stroke 26:2184–2186
26. Georgiadis D, Goeke J, Stögbauer F, et al (1996) A novel technique for identification of Doppler microembolic signals based on the coincidence method. In vitro and in vivo evaluation. Stroke 27:683–686
27. Babikian VI, Droste DW, Evans DH, et al (1998) Consensus statement on microembolus detection by transcranial Doppler ultrasound. Stroke (submitted)
28. Weiller C, Ringelstein EB, Reiche W, Thron A, Buell U (1990) The large striatocapsular infarct. A clinical and pathophysiological entity. Arch Neurol 47:1085–1091
29. Wong KS, Liang EY, Lam WW, Huang YN, Kay R (1995) Spiral computed tomography angiography in the assessment of middle cerebral artery occlusive disease. J Neurol Neurosurg Psychiat 59:537–539
30. Hacke W, Kaste M, Fieschi C, et al (1995) Intravenous thrombolysis with recombinant tissue plasminogen activator for acute hemispheric stroke. JAMA 274:1017–1025
31. Zanette EM, Roberti C, Mancini G, Pozzilli C, Bragoni M, Toni D (1995) Spontaneous middle cerebral artery reperfusion in ischemic stroke. A follow-up study with transcranial Doppler. Stroke 26:430–433
32. Kaps M, Teschendorf U, Dorndorf W (1992) Hemodynamic studies in early stroke. J Neurol 239:138–142
33. Kaps M, Link A (1997) Transcranial ultrasound monitoring during thrombolytic therapy. Am J Neuroradiol (in press)
34. Pulsinelli W (1992) Pathophysiology of acute ischaemic stroke. Lancet 339:16–19
35. Fieschi C, Argentino C, Lenai GL, et al (1989) Clinical and instrumental evaluation of patients with ischemic stroke within the first six hours. J Neurolg Sci 91:311–321
36. Baron JC, Frackowiak RSJ, Herholz K, et al (1989) Use of positron emission tomography in the investigation of cerebral hemodynamics and energy metabolism in cerebrovascular disease. J Cereb Blood Flow Metab 9:723–742
37. Gibbs JM, Wise RJS, Leenders KL, et al (1984) Evaluation of cerebral perfusion reserve in patients with carotid-artery occlusion. Lancet:310–314
38. Sette G, Baron JC, Mazoyer B, et al (1989), Local brain hemodynamics and oxygen metabolism in cerebrovascular disease: positron emission tomography. Brain 112:931–951
39. Baron JC, Rougemont D, Sousaline F, et al (1984) Local interrelationship of cerebral oxygen consumption and glucose utilization in normal subjects and in ischemic stroke patients: a positron tomography study. J Cereb Blood Flow Metab 4:140–149
40. Baron JC, Samson Y, Pantano P, et al (1987) Inter relationships of local CBF, OEF and CMRO2 in ischemic areas with variable outcome: further PET studies in humans. J Cereb Blood Flow Metab (suppl 1):41
41. Powers WJ, Grubb RL Jr, Darriet D, et al (1985) Cerebral blood flow and cerebral metabolic rate of oxygen requirements for cerebral function and viability in humans. J Cereb Blood Flow Metab 5:500–608
42. Ackerman RH, Lev MH, Mackay BC, et al (1989) PET studies in acute stroke: Findings and relevance to therapy. J Cereb Blood Flow Metab 9 (suppl 1):S359
43. Wise RJS, Bernardi S, Frackowiak RSJ, et al (1983) Serial observations on the pathophysiology of acute stroke. The transition from ischaemia to infarction as reflected in regional oxygen extraction. Brain 106:197–222
44. Marchal G, Serrati C, Rioux P, et al (1993) PET imaging of cerebral perfusion and oxygen consumption in acute ischaemic stroke: relation to outcome. Lancet 341:925–927
45. Marchal G, Rioux P, Beaudoin V, et al (1995a) Severe hypoperfusion/hypometabolism in acute stroke: an index of the minimum extent of irreversible damage. Cerebrovas Dis 5:230
46. Marchal G, Furlan M, Beaudoin V, et al (1996a) Early spontaneous hyperperfusion after stroke: a marker of favorable tissue outcome. Brain 119:409–419
47. Heiss WD, Huber M, Fink GR, et al (1992) Progressive derangement of periinfarct viable tissue in ischemic stroke. J Cereb Blood Flow Metab 12:193–203

48. Marchal G, Beaudouin V, Rioux P, et al (1996b) Prolonged persistence of substantial volume of potentially viable brain tissue after stroke: a correlate PET-CT study with voxel-based data analysis. Stroke 27:599–606
49. Marchal G, Rioux P, Serrati C, et al (1995b) Value of acute-stage PET in predicting neurological outcome after ischemic stroke: further assessment. Stroke 26:524–525
50. Furlan M, Marchal G, Viader F, et al (1996) Spontaneous neurological recovery after stroke and the fate of the ischemic penumbra Ann Neurology 40:216–226
51. Jorgensen H, Nakayama H, Raaschou HO, et al (1994) Effect of blood pressure and diabetes on stroke in progression. Lancet 344:156–159

Modern Imaging Technology in the Assessment of Acute Ischemic Stroke

R. E. Latchaw and M. Fisher

Introduction

Advances in modern imaging techniques are being applied in two areas of acute stroke management: refining triage decisions on which patients should receive thrombolytic therapy, and improving clinical trials of new stroke treatments. For guiding thrombolytic therapy decisions, the need is to be able to determine whether there is sufficient salvageable tissue to warrant the risks of treatment. These risks include reperfusion injury and hemorrhagic complications.

There is also a need for surrogate endpoints in stroke trials. Clinical endpoints have wide variability (as in lacunar vs cortical lesions) and require large numbers of patients, increasing the expense and time required for clinical studies. The ideal surrogate endpoint for stroke trials would be easily and rapidly obtainable, of reasonable cost, exclude inappropriate or untreatable patients, determine lesion size before and after treatment, and, of course, be acceptable to regulatory agencies. The goal of surrogate endpoints is not to replace clinical endpoints but to speed up the development of therapies and to provide alternative *in vivo* markers of therapeutic responses. Diffusion-perfusion MRI is probably as close to the ideal as is now possible.

Physiological Principles

The reversibility of ischemia is dependent upon both the level of cerebral blood flow (CBF) and the duration of the ischemic process. As regional CBF falls below 20 ml/100 g/min, neuronal activity ceases. Tissue receiving CBF ranging from 10 to 20 ml/100 g/min require a longer period of ischemia before irreversible infarction occurs than tissue having CBF of less than 10 ml/100 g/min, in which infarction occurs within minutes (Fig. 1) [1]. Collateral circulation provides greater CBF on the periphery (the penumbra) of a central core of more profound ischemia (Fig. 2). The central core might already be infarcted when the patient is seen, but the penumbra may contain salvageable tissue (Fig. 3). Thus, the question of whether to undertake therapies to rescue the brain is not answered by evaluating only the time after the onset of the stroke. Rather, the essential question is how much viable tissue remains, whatever the time factor.

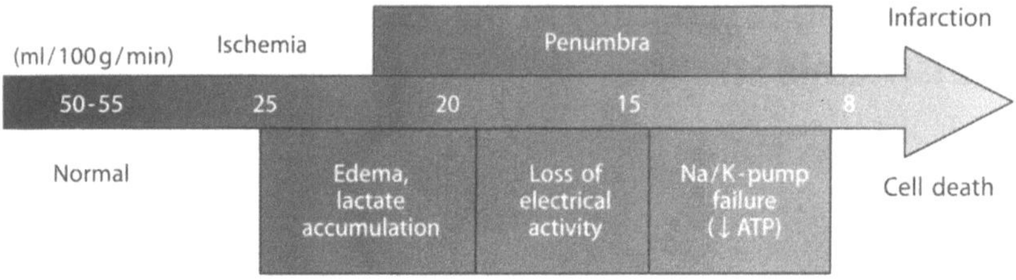

Fig. 1. Effects of reduced cerebral blood flow. As the level of blood flow decreases, there are progressive tissue changes leading to infarction. (Figure courtesy of the National Stroke Association)

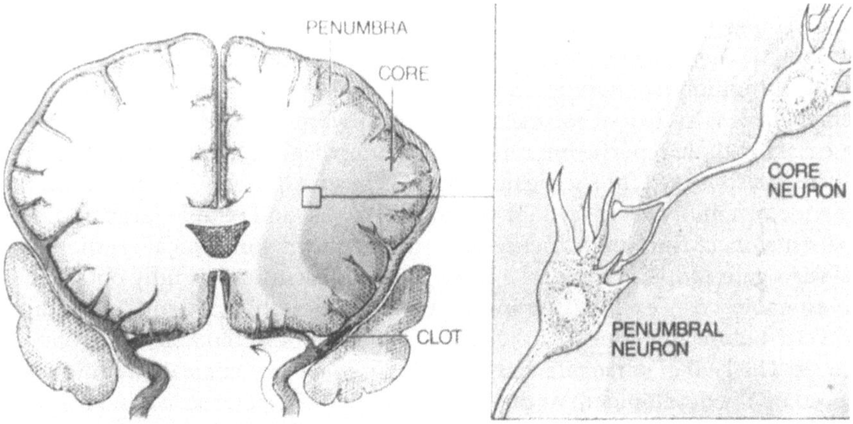

Fig. 2. Schematic diagram of the penumbra. Around the central core of infarction, there is an area (the penumbra) in which collateral circulation keeps the ischemic tissue viable for a period of time

Clinical Questions

Current management options during the first few hours after stroke onset include medical management (with or without the use of heparin), intravenous neuroprotective agents, intravenous administration of thrombolytic agents, and the intra-arterial administration of thrombolytics. Can the potential for tissue salvation be estimated by determining the amount of brain that is ischemic but not yet infarcted? Should thrombolytics be used if most of the ischemic brain is already dead?

The risk of reperfusion injury following thrombolysis, particularly hemorrhagic transformation of the infarct and hematoma formation, is a significant concern. Is the risk of using a thrombolytic agent unacceptably high if there is a large area of infarcted tissue present? Can the risk of reperfusion injury be estimated by determining the ratio of salvageable to nonsalvageable tissue?

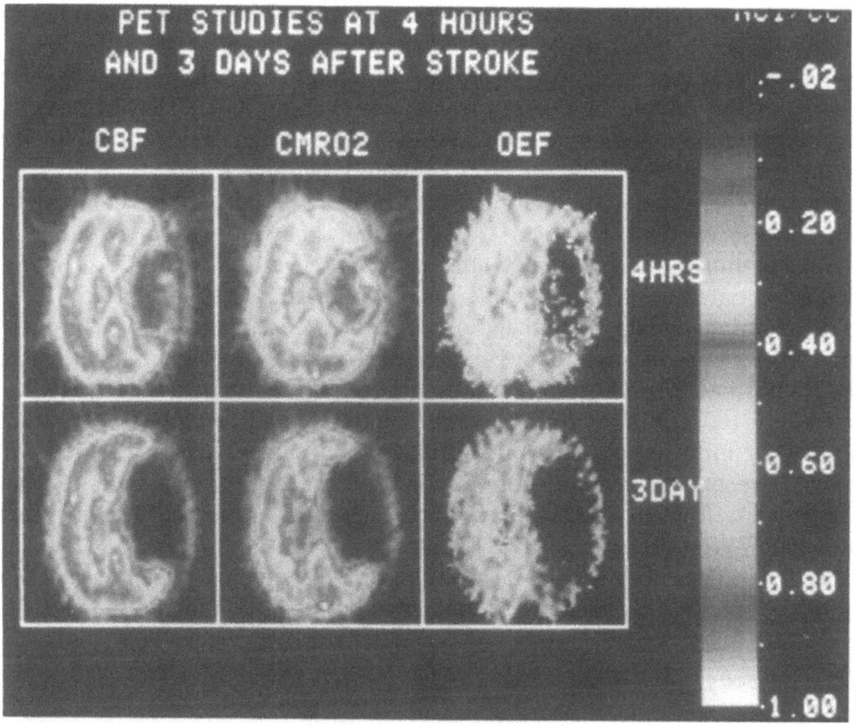

Fig. 3. PET studies demonstrating the penumbra at the time of acute stroke and its loss over time. The positron emission tomographic studies demonstrate the penumbra (blue) surrounding the central core of infarction (black) on the CBF study. No thrombolytic therapy was provided, and by three days the infarction had extended to include the penumbra. (Figure courtesy of Dr. Robert Ackerman, Massachusetts General Hospital)

Thus, there is a need to identify and to quantify the amount of salvageable brain in order to (1) insure the diagnosis of acute ischemia, (2) help determine prognosis, (3) estimate the risk of complications, and (4) serve as a tool to make management decisions.

Imaging methods for detecting and evaluating the salvageable brain include those based on computed tomography (CT perfusion, CT angiography, xenon/CT cerebral blood flow analysis), magnetic resonance imaging (diffusion, perfusion, MR angiography, spectroscopy), and nuclear medicine studies (SPECT cerebral blood flow analysis, positron emission tomography).

CT Techniques in Stroke

The nonenhanced CT scan is useful for excluding intracranial hemorrhage which is a contraindication for the use of drugs for thrombolysis or anticoagulation. The early signs of ischemia may also be seen, which include the following: (1)

decreased contrast differentiation between gray and white matter structures, including the deep basal ganglia and adjacent white matter tracks, the insular cortical ribbon, and the corticomedullary junctions over the cortex; (2) sulcal effacement and ventricular compression due to swelling; and (3) lowered density of gray and white matter structures. The sooner these signs are seen and the larger the area of involvement, the more profound the degree and extent of ischemia, which correlates with a poorer outcome and a higher risk for hemorrhage with the use of thrombolytics [2]. These signs may be extremely subtle or invisible within the first few hours after stroke onset, and the plain CT scan does not differentiate between salvageable and nonsalvageable ischemic brain.

CT scanning during the inhalation of stable xenon produces quantitative blood flow maps that can define an area of ischemia when the plain CT scan appears normal. It can also differentiate between those areas that have CBF less than 10 ml/100 g/min, and are therefore infarcted, and areas between 10 and 20 ml/100 g/min that are ischemic but potentially salvageable (Fig. 4) [3]. The xenon/CT technique requires only 4 minutes of inhalation of a xenon-oxygen mixture and 10 minutes of computer processing time, and can be performed immediately after the emergency CT study.

The hyperdense middle cerebral artery sign gives evidence of the presence of a thrombus, but it is only present in about 30% of cases [4]. CT angiography (CTA)

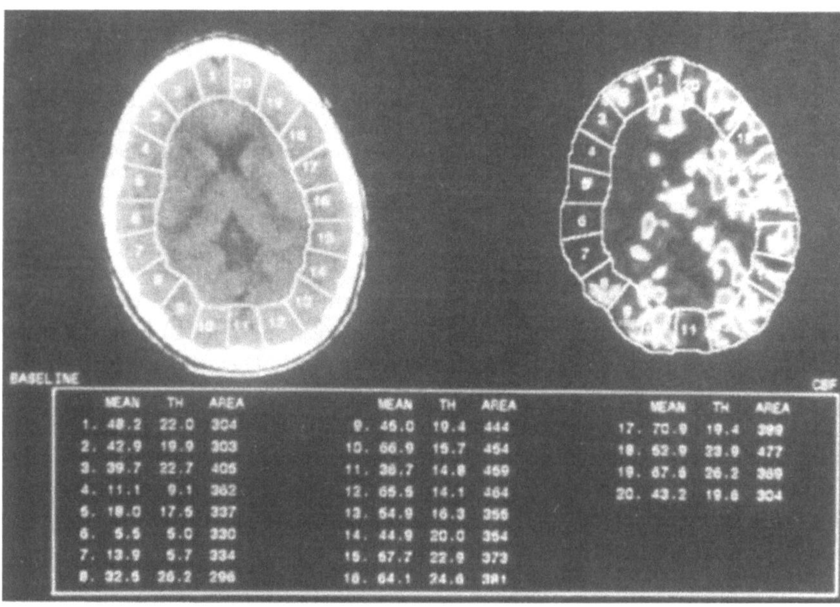

Fig. 4. Xenon-CT demonstrating right MCA acute stroke with variable blood flow values. In this patient with acute stroke, the plain CT scan on the left is normal, while the CBF study with Xenon demonstrates the low flows in the right middle cerebral distribution. This quantitative technique demonstrates low flows in the regions of interest numbered 4 through 7, having CBF values ranging from 5.5 to 18.0 cc/100gm/min. At the lower values, the tissue is almost surely infarcted, while at the upper ranges, the tissue is probably viable

can give very detailed anatomic information regarding the presence of an intravascular thrombus, facilitating a decision to be made for the use of intravenous or intra-arterial thrombolytic drugs (Fig. 5) [5]. The technique requires the intravenous injection of 90 ml of a contrast agent and rapid helical scanning through the base of the brain. Faster computer processing times and larger scanning volumes are developments making this an increasingly popular technique to evaluate all forms of cerebrovascular disease.

Perfusion CT evaluates the transit time for the contrast bolus to pass through the cerebral vasculature during helical CT scanning, and could be performed as part of the CTA procedure [6]. The need to assess the efficacy of therapy while it is being given, particularly intra-arterial thrombolysis, suggests the possibility of a hybrid CT scanner/angiography suite. After the patient has been evaluated in the emergency room and moved to the CT/angiography suite, the pre-thrombolytic studies could include plain CT, CTA, and perfusion CT and/or xenon/CT. Thrombolysis is started, and therapy is guided by repeating the physiological studies.

MR in Acute Stroke

Standard spin-echo and gradient-echo MR imaging does not consistently demonstrate the parenchymal abnormalities of ischemia early enough to be useful in the triage of a patient for acute therapy. Contrast-enhanced MR demonstrates enhancement of vessels beyond an obstruction that are usually hypointense because of rapidly flowing blood [7]. However, this is not a consistent sign because a high grade obstruction produces poor filling of the vessels in question by the collateral circulation. Finally, none of these MR techniques differentiates between

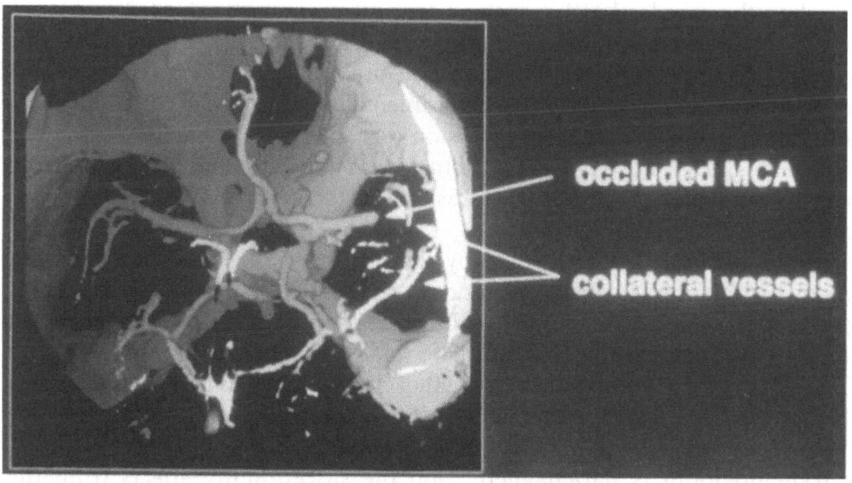

Fig. 5. CTA demonstrating occluded left middle cerebral artery. (Figure courtesy of Dr. Werner Hacke and Dr. Klaus Sartor, Heidelberg, Germany)

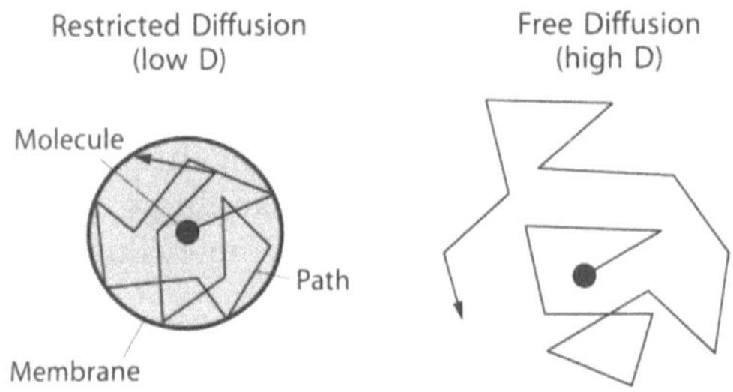

Fig. 6. Diagram of restricted diffusion (left) versus free diffusion (right)

reversible and nonreversible ischemia in the first few hours after insult. However, newer MR techniques such as diffusion and perfusion MR appear capable of demonstrating the ischemic region within minutes to hours after its onset and of defining the salvageable brain.

Diffusion weighted MR studies are obtained by using very powerful gradient coils that are capable of undergoing rapid switches in polarity. Diffusion in the presence of these gradient pulses produces incoherent phase shifts, so that the relative rate of movement of water molecules can be determined. Membranes and myelin sheaths produce natural impediments to diffusion. Further restriction of the movement of water occurs when it encounters the intracellular environment of macromolecules and organelle membranes (Fig. 6). As the CBF falls and cells become ischemic, the cell membrane allows sodium and water to flow from the extracellular to the intracellular space, producing cytotoxic edema. This results in a decrease in the overall diffusion coefficients in the ischemic region. Diffusion can be measured quantitatively in the X, Y, and Z directions; apparent diffusion coefficients (ADC's) can be determined. Diffusion MR may show abnormalities within minutes after an ischemic insult, allowing a diagnosis of an ischemic insult when the standard MR sequences are still normal [8]. The T-2 spin-echo sequence, so sensitive to the presence of vasogenic edema, becomes abnormal later, reflecting the abnormality to the blood-brain barrier. The accuracy of diffusion MR was demonstrated in an experimental animal model of stroke using middle cerebral artery occlusion. Diffusion was abnormal at one hour after the occlusion (Fig. 7A) although the T2 study was normal (Fig. 7B). The tissue damage in the region of abnormal diffusion was confirmed by the pathological specimen (Fig. 7C).

Perfusion MR can be performed by detecting the magnetic susceptibility effects of paramagnetic substances on protons surrounding capillaries. A paramagnetic contrast agent is injected and the decreased signal from the perfused tissues is demonstrated over time using a rapid MR sequence that is sensitive to the T-2* effect of the contrast [9]. Arterial occlusion leads to less perfusion, less signal decrease, and hence ischemic tissue appears more intense relative to the less intense normal tissues (Fig. 8).

Deoxyhemoglobin is paramagnetic, and the susceptibility effects from the subject's own blood, reflecting CBF, is the basis for another technique of functional MR imaging [10]. Useful information can be obtained from curves deriv-

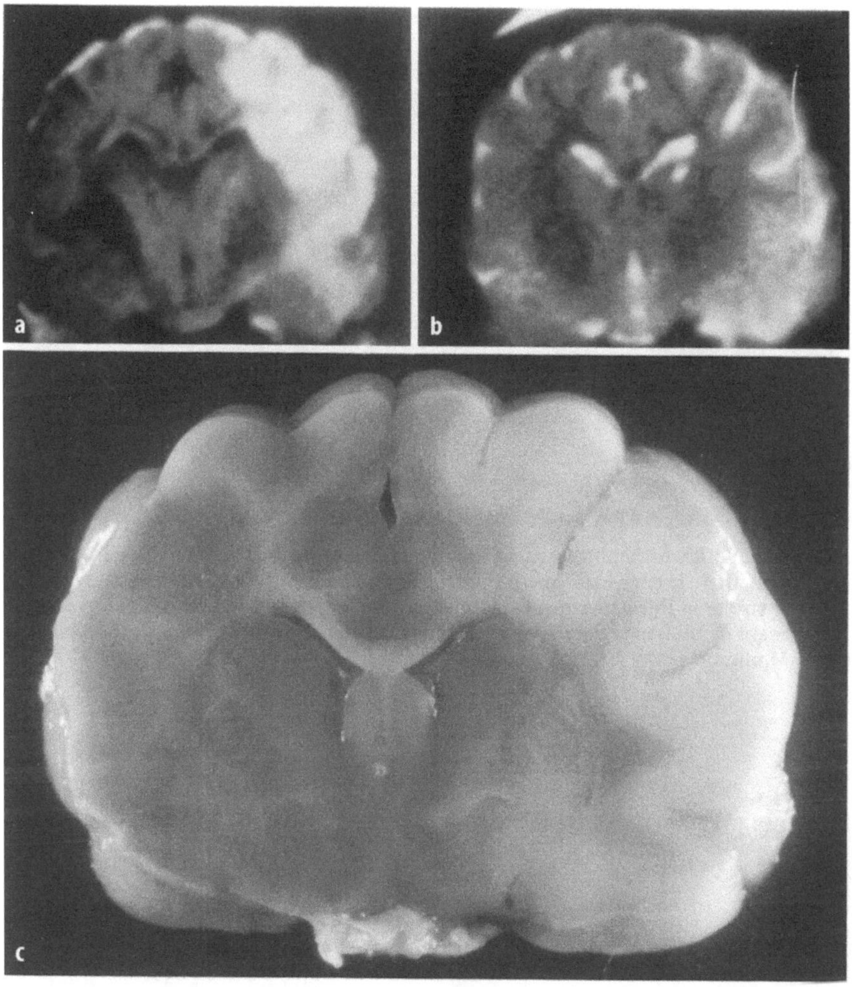

Fig. 7. Left MCA occlusion in experimental animal imaged with diffusion MR. The left MCA has been occluded in this experimental animal, with diffusion imaging at one hour. On the left (**A**), the left MCA distribution is hyperintense, characteristic of decreased diffusion from ischemia. On the right (**B**) the T-2 weighted MR study at the same time is unremarkable. The pathological specimen (**C**) confirms the abnormality seen on the diffusion study (**A**). (Figures courtesy of Dr. John Kucharczyk, University of Minnesota)

ed from the kinetics of the contrast agent flow to demonstrate blood volumes, mean transit time, and delay in the bolus speed. It may be possible to quantify this information to use the blood volume and mean transit time to derive CBF [9].

There are questions about whether diffusion MRI shows both reversible and nonreversible ischemia or represents only infarction. In clinical practice it may be that the diffusion abnormality represents dead tissue. This makes it possible to

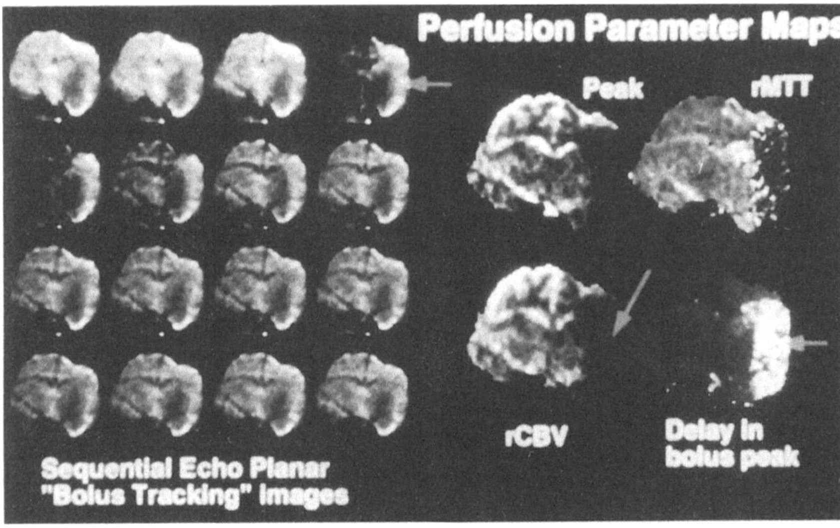

Fig. 8. Perfusion MR with "bolus tracking" technique. Following the injection of a paramagnetic contrast agent, there is decreased intensity of the brain tissue in the areas of normal perfusion. The area of stroke in this experimental animal remains hyperintense (left MCA). A variety of perfusion maps demonstrate the area of ischemia. (Figure courtesy of Dr. John Kucharczyk, University of Minnesota)

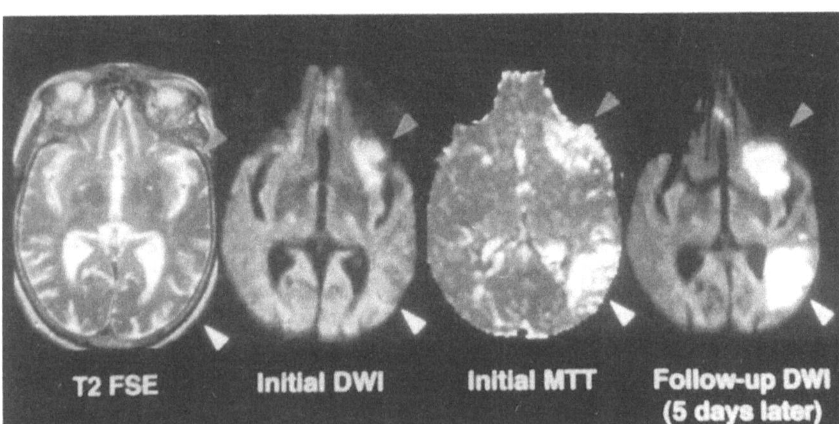

Fig. 9. Acute stroke diffusion/perfusion mismatch. In this patient with stroke only a few hours old, the T-2-weighted MR study is normal, and the diffusion-weighted sequence shows a relatively small abnormality in the anterior left temporal region. However, the perfusion (MTT, mean transit time) map shows two large areas of perfusion abnormality. No thrombolytic treatment was given, and five days later the diffusion abnormalities equal the perfusion defects, indicating that the tissue which was at risk has now become infarcted. (Figure courtesy of Dr. Gilberto Gonzalez, Massachusetts General Hospital)

use the diffusion-perfusion mismatch to differentiate the penumbral tissue (the territory at risk with lowered perfusion) from the central core of infarction (Fig. 9) [11]. The ultimate test of this hypothesis would be to do diffusion-perfusion MRI before and after thrombolysis in a large series of patients. The ideal setting would be thrombolysis performed on an MR system to monitor therapy, and imaging systems combining MR and fluoroscopy are being developed.

It is important that there is a reliable vascular screening test to demonstrate if a patient has a major vessel occlusion in order to decide who should receive a thrombolytic agent, and who might benefit from intra-arterial catheterization for clot lysis and removal. Such therapies are expensive, and accurate screening is essential. A CT-based scenario, using CTA for such screening, has already been described, but a MR-based scenario, using MRA, would also be feasible (Fig. 10) [12]. A patient might go directly from the emergency room to the MR suite for MRI, MRA, perfusion and diffusion MR; thrombolysis performed on the magnet as indicated; and the MR studies repeated. Such a scenario requires the ability to visualize intracranial blood in the acute stage, and new pulsing sequences appear promising for this need [13].

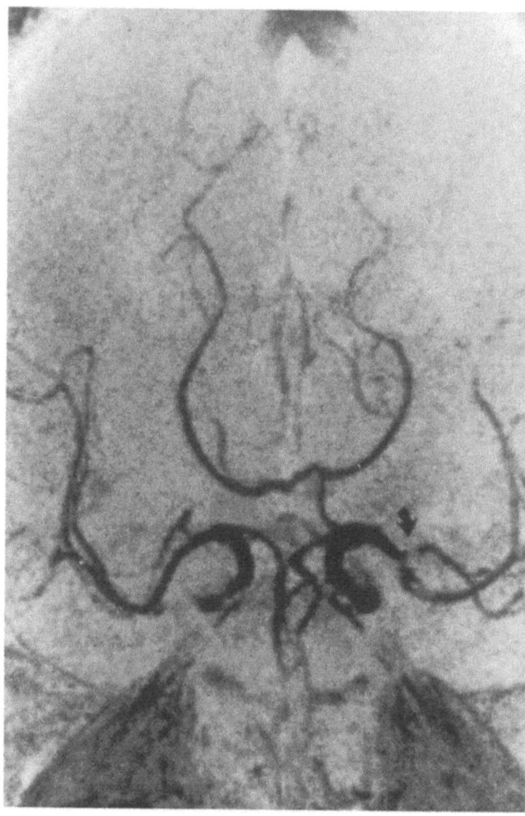

Fig. 10. MRA of the circle of Willis demonstrating an embolus in the distal aspect of the left middle cerebral artery (arrow)

Evolution of Ischemic Lesions Over Time

Animal models have been helpful in defining the evolution of ischemic lesions over time. Animal studies of lesion size evolution using a suture occlusion model in rats showed that at two and three hours after occlusion the lesion had maximized and was highly correlated with postmortem infarct volume (Fig. 11) [14]. Studies with the NMDA antagonist Cerestat in this model showed a substantial difference in ischemic lesion size [15]. The lesion size was essentially frozen at the size defined by MRI at the time of treatment for animals receiving rt-PA (Fig. 12). In another experiment, postmortem studies showed a significant difference in

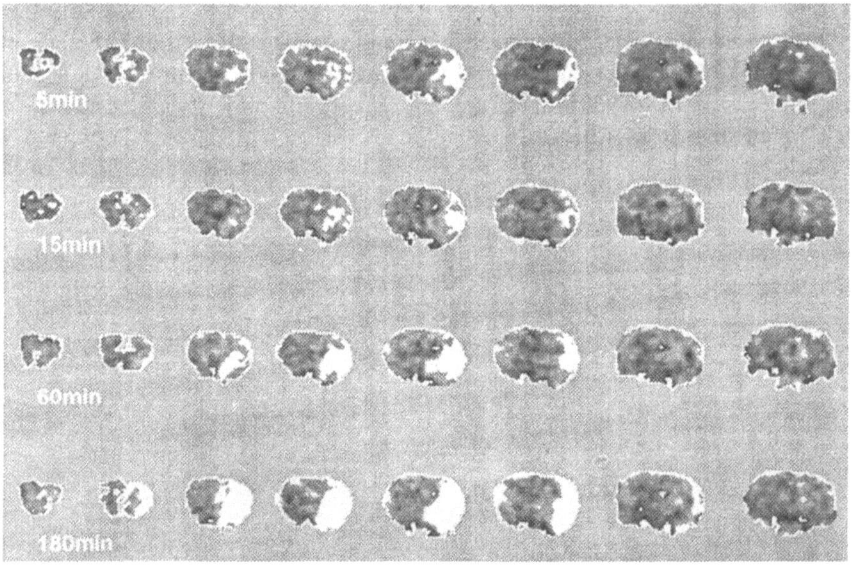

Fig. 11. Evolution of lesion size in the rat model. By two to three hours after suture occlusion, the lesion had maximized and was highly correlated with postmortem infarct volume

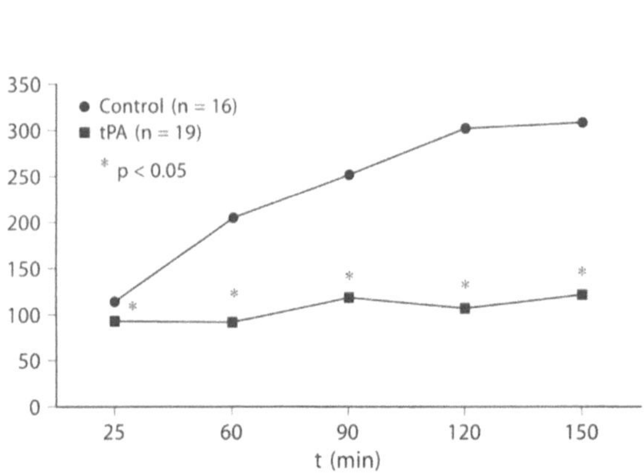

Fig. 12. Effect of Cerestat on the evolving lesion. The lesion was essentially stabilized at the time of treatment

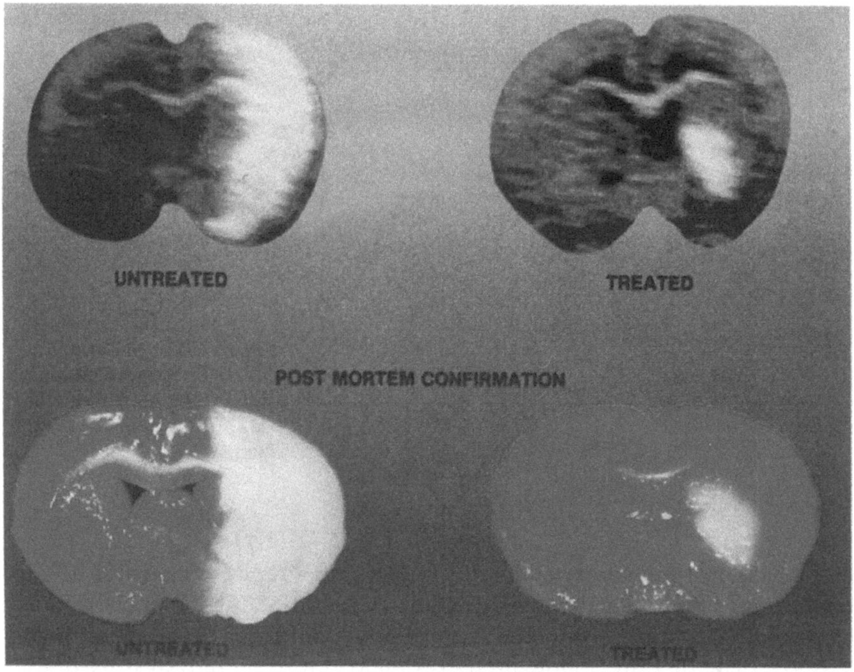

Fig. 13. Postmortem study of Cerestat-treated animal. Postmortem studies showed a significant difference in infarct size in treated versus untreated animals

infarct size in the treated animals (Fig. 13). Combining Cerestat with reperfusion at three hours showed that reperfusion significantly reduced infarct size in the treated animals (Fig. 14). This suggests that drugs such as Cerestat might extend the treatment window in acute stroke. Realizing the process of neuroprotection will require a more complete understanding and imaging of ischemic lesions and their changes over time.

Evolution of the lesion is slower in humans than in animal models [16]. Serial scanning at 4, 28, and 56 hours after right MCA occlusion demonstrates slower expansion of the infarct within the penumbra than might be anticipated (Fig. 15). In a series of patients with acute stroke, the lesion volume increased by more than 20% in 12 of 15 patients between 6 hours after onset and 6–12 weeks after onset [17]. In many patients the evolution of lesion size is much slower than was thought. This supports a need to individualize treatment, not just assume that all stroke patients have 3-hour treatment window [18]. One way to do this is to rely on MRI images to define tissue at risk for ischemic damage.

In using diffusion-perfusion MRI to assess therapy, pretreatment studies should be compared to delayed T2 images. The evolution of ischemic lesion volume over time will likely be the primary analysis. Therapeutic effects on the MRI parameters should be correlated with clinical efficacy. Minimally, baseline pretreatment diffusion-perfusion MRI and a T2 study should be taken, there

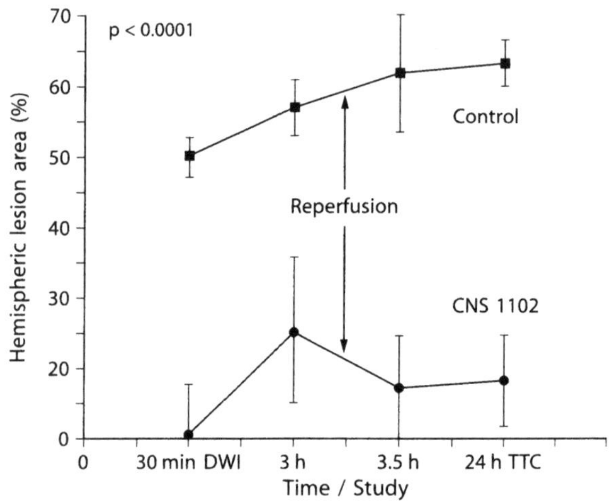

Fig. 14. Effect of Cerestat plus reperfusion. Combining treatment with reperfusion significantly reduced the infarct size

should be a follow-up battery at day 30–90, MR angiography should also be considered prior to treatment. These MRI studies can be obtained in approximately 30 minutes. The possible design for a clinical trial would thus be: baseline clinical MRI study; drug therapy; follow-up perfusion MRI if thrombolysis is used; routine clinical assessments; and 30–90 day MRI studies.

Diffusion-perfusion MRI may facilitate other tasks in addition to measuring lesions volumes. These include assessing stroke subtypes, documenting perfusion deficits, evaluating therapeutic responses, and perhaps documenting the existence of potentially salvageable tissue so that patients without any can be excluded from clinical trials. With information about the timing and progression of human stroke, diffusion-perfusion MRI may also aid individualization of treatment "time windows."

A reasonable intra-arterial thrombolysis scenario using MR might be: MRI and MR angiography; perfusion/diffusion MRI; thrombolysis on the magnet with real-time imaging; and MRI, MRA or perfusion MRI after the thrombolytic drug is finished.

Conclusion

The new imaging technologies are expected to have a significant impact on the evaluation and treatment of acute stroke, particularly as we enter the era of multiple therapies. Neuroprotective therapies such as NMDA antagonists might be used very early, perhaps even in the ambulance, followed by thrombolysis in patients who have appropriate clinical deficits after this early therapy and who show perfusion deficits or an occluded artery on imaging studies. Alternatively, where MRI demonstrates the absence of a perfusion deficit, the next step might be antiadhesion molecules or antioxidants.

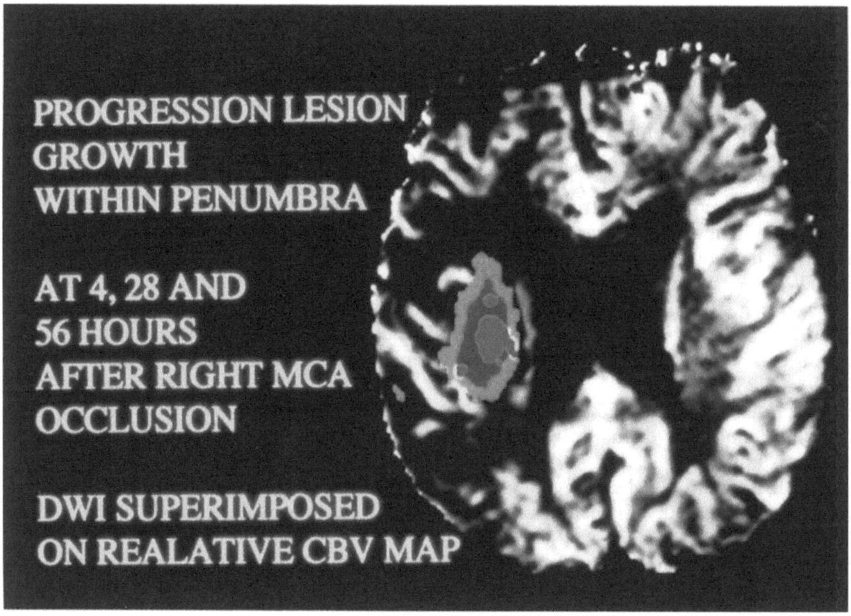

Fig. 15. Progression of lesions in humans. Serial scanning after right MCA occlusion suggests that the expansion of the infarct within the penumbra is slower than might be anticipated. This demonstrates the importance of not assuming that all stroke patients have a 3-hour treatment window

References

1. Heiss WD, Rosner G (1983) Functional recovery of cortical neurons as related to degree and duration of ischemia. Ann Neurol 14:294–301
2. von Kummer R, Meyding-Lamade U, Forsting M et al (1994) Sensitivity and prognostic value of early CT in occlusion of the middle cerebral artery trunk. Am J Neuroradiol 15:9–15
3. Yonas H, Gur D, Latchaw RE, Wolfson SK (1987) Xenon computed tomographic blood flow mapping. In : Wood JH (ed) Cerebral blood flow: physiologic and clinical aspects. McGraw-Hill Co., New York, pp 220–242
4. Tomsick TA, Brott TG, Chambers AA, et al (1990) Hyperdense middle cerebral artery sign on CT: efficacy in detecting middle cerebral artery thrombosis. Am J Neuroradiol 11:473–477
5. Shrier DA, Tanaka H, Numaguchi Y, Konno S, Patel U, Shibata D (1997) CT angiography in the evaluation of acute stroke. Am J Neuroradiol 18:1011–1020
6. Hamberg LM, Hunter GJ, Kierstead D, Lo EH, Gonzalez RG, Wolf GL (1996) Measurement of cerebral blood volume with subtraction three-dimensional functional CT. Am J Neuroradiol 17:1861–1869
7. Yuh WTC, Crain MR, Loes DJ, Greene GM, Ryals TJ, Sato Y (1991) MR imaging of cerebral ischemia: findings in the first 24 hours. Am J Neuroradiol 12:621–629
8. Mosely ME, Kucharczyk J, Mintorovitch J, et al (1990) Diffusion-weighted MR imaging of acute stroke: correlation with T2-weighted and magnetic susceptibility-enhanced MR imaging in cats. Am J Neuroradiol 11:423–429
9. Kucharczyk J, Vexler ZS, Roberts TP, et al (1993) Echo-planar perfusion-sensitive MR imaging of acute cerebral ischemia. Radiology 188:711–717

10. Latchaw RE, Hu X, Ugurbil K, Hall WA, Madison MT, Heros RC (1995) Functional magnetic resonance imaging as a management tool for cerebral arteriovenous malformations. Neurosurgery 37:619–626
11. Sorenson AG, Buonanno FS, Gonzalez RG, et al (1996) Hyperacute stroke: evaluation with combined multisection diffusion-weighted and hemodynamically weighted echo-planar MR imaging. Radiology 199:391–401
12. Furst G, Hofer M, Steinmetz H, et al (1996) Intracranial stenoocclusive disease: MR angiography with magnetization transfer and variable flip angle. Am J Neuroradiol 17:1749–1757
13. Patel MR, Edelman RR, Warach S (1996) Detection of hyperacute primary intraparenchymal hemorrhage by magnetic resonance imaging. Stroke 27:2321–2324
14. Relts W, Hasegawa Y, Latour U. et al (1995) Multislice diffusion mapping for 3–0 evolution of cerebral ischemia in a rat stroke model. Neurology 45:172–177
15. Mineratsu K, Fisher MLL, Sotak CH (1993) Diffusion and perfusion MRI studies to evaluate a non-competitive NMDA antagonist and reperfusion in experimental stroke. Stroke 24:2074–2081
16. Sorensen AB, Buonanno FS, Gonzalez RB, et al (1996) Hyperacute stroke: evaluation with combined multislice diffusion-weighted and hemodynamically weighted echoplanar MRI imaging. Radiology 199:391–401
17. Baird AE, Benfield A, Sclaug G, et al (1997) Enlargement of human cerebral ischemic lesion volumes measured by diffusion-weighted magnetic resonance imaging. Ann Neurol 41:581–589
18. Baron JC, von Kummar R, del Zoppo GJ (1995) Treatment of acute ischemic stroke: challenging the concept of a rigid and universal time window. Stroke 26:2219–2221

Thrombolytic Therapy in Acute Ischemic Stroke

J. R. Marler, C. Fieschi, R. Higashida, and G. Boysen

Introduction

Data from two large multi-center studies show that thrombolysis can improve outcomes in some patients with acute ischemic stroke. Hemorrhage remains a concern, as does finding ways to increase the proportion of patients who respond to treatment. To be effective, clot lysis must be accompanied by re-establishing local perfusion of viable brain tissue. New technical developments will facilitate the application of intra-arterial thrombolysis and angioplasty for these purposes. More research is needed into the factors which predict good or bad responses to thrombolysis and into clot composition and hemodynamic flow dynamics.

Thrombolysis after the NINDS and ECASS Studies: Where Do We Go Now?

The major clinical goals with regard to acute ischemic stroke are to prevent the stroke or, when prevention fails, to treat stroke quickly to limit disability. Although there were differences between the European Cooperative Acute Stroke Study (ECASS) and the U.S. National Institute of Neurological Disease and Stroke rt-PA Stroke Study Group (NINDS) trials, there are also areas of agreement [1, 2]. The most important is clear evidence that acute intervention in stroke can improve outcomes in some patients. That is a new and exciting finding. Both trials also found that early treatment and careful patient selection are important and that not all patients will respond to the current regimen.

The ECASS and NINDS trials were successful because of the careful way in which all the major steps in drug development were followed:

- Preclinical Laboratory Research
- Phase 1 Dose Determination Studies
- Phase 2 Estimates of Efficacy
- Phase 3 Trials of Effectiveness
- Analysis of Results
- Changing Standard Clinical Care
- New Preclinical Research Problems

We are now in the phase of analyzing results and generating new preclinical basic laboratory research problems to address.

Several pilot studies preceded the NINDS and ECASS trials. One separated patients into those treated within 0–90 minutes after symptom onset and those treated at 91–180 minutes. Those studies showed an increase in favorable response for earlier treatment, with a decrease in hemorrhage [3, 4]. This lead to design of the Phase 2 and Phase 3 trials.

However, the overall finding of these two trials is that, depending on analysis criteria, 50% to 69% of patients did not improve after thrombolysis. This may have been because treatment was too late, because treatment was not able to dissolve the clot, or because hemorrhage obscured the treatment benefit. Further development of stroke treatments is needed.

Future trials should be designed to increase the number of eligible patients, reduce hemorrhage, and include new treatments that will increase the proportion of responders. Increasing the number of eligible patients requires changing medical practice so that patients can be treated earlier. We should also explore the benefits from longer time windows for entry.

Recanalization can occur at any time (Fig. 1). However, the brain's ability to respond diminishes over time and probably varies by individual and by other characteristics related to collateral circulation and to interventions such as the treatment of blood pressure. The risk of other complications increases over time. Thrombolysis thus has benefits up to a certain point but can be harmful later. It is very likely that any successful treatment will be more beneficial if it can be given sooner.

Reducing the hemorrhage rate is likely to require lower doses of thrombolytic agents, more selective lytic agents, more research on the mechanism underlying thrombolysis-induced intracerebral hemorrhage, and more stringent control of blood pressure.

Increasing the response rate may require new thrombolytic agents, earlier treatment, and combination therapy with other agents that enhance collateral circulation or increase ischemia tolerance by reducing metabolic demands and/or delaying destructive metabolic processes.

A number of unanswered questions remain. One is the composition of the clots that cause strokes. Another is the mechanism by which thrombolytic agents

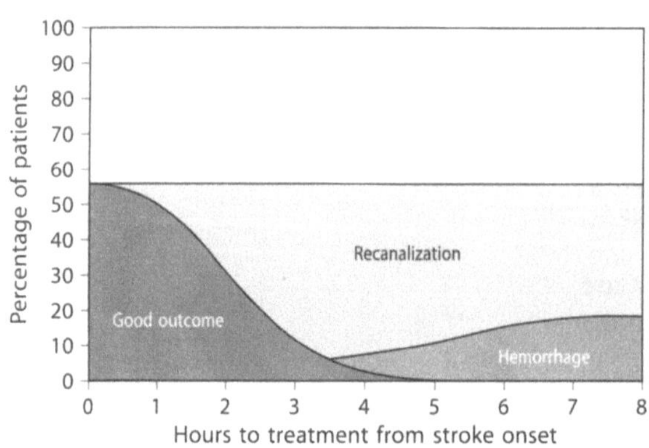

Fig. 1. Time determines possible benefit

cause intracranial hemorrhage. The final is how to increase the early recognition of stroke by the general population.

Non-pharmacological therapy should not be overlooked. Mechanical disruption of the clot can involve disruption by a catheter, external ultrasound, and efforts to reverse flow. Hypothermia has been described as the gold standard of neuroprotection [4], but it is difficult to apply and seldom practicable. Establishing the level of consciousness at 33 degrees C is difficult. Conscious patients are likely to shiver so much they will need sedation. Patients are more likely to develop infection. Hypothermia is tremendously stressful for older patients. Finally, it affects hemostasis and has unknown effects on the rate of thrombolysis. Many challenges remain.

Future efforts should be directed at changing medical care to increase the number of patients available for early treatment. We should also increase research on the mechanisms of brain hemorrhage due to thrombolysis, identify subgroups of patients according to etiology, study clot composition, and support pilot studies of combined therapy where a brain-protective agent may be administered out-of-hospital. There are so many promising neuroprotective treatments and strategies that the race to find a better treatment for acute stroke will eventually succeed.

New Aspects of the ECASS Trial

Despite an increased incidence of intracerebral hemorrhage, an improvement in clinical outcome at three months was found in patients in the ECASS study treated with intravenous rt-PA within six hours of the onset of acute ischemic stroke. However, both ECASS and a recent European Ad Hoc Consensus Statement agree that intravenous thrombolysis is beneficial only in selected patients with acute ischemic stroke, not in an unselected population of patients [5].

In the ECASS trial 92 patients were treated at less than 3 hours (40 placebo, 52 rt-PA) [6]. In this early treatment group there was a 25% increase in fatalities but a 62% increase in patients with good outcomes (Rankin 0–1) (Fig. 2). Altogether, treatment seems to be advantageous at this time. In patients treated after 3 hours, there was a 40% increase in fatalities with only a slight (17%) increase in good outcomes (Fig. 3).

Initial computed tomography (CT) showed a higher percentage of early hypodensity in ECASS compared to NINDS patients (Fig. 4). The ECASS patients also had significantly more brain swelling and more parenchymal hemorrhage after treatment (Fig. 5). These differences may reflect differences in the dose of rt-PA or the severity of neurological deficit.

The first implication for future trials is that patients with extended early CT signs should be excluded from trials of thrombolysis, regardless of the interval between stroke onset and hospitalization. This raises the question of whether early CT signs are always an index of irreversible damage. A related question is whether patients with extended early CT signs should participate in randomized trials with antiedema agents?

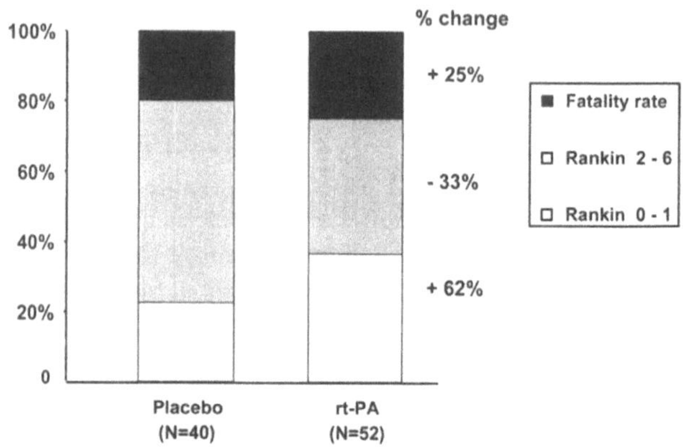

Fig. 2. ECASS trial: Clinical outcome of patients treated before 3 hours

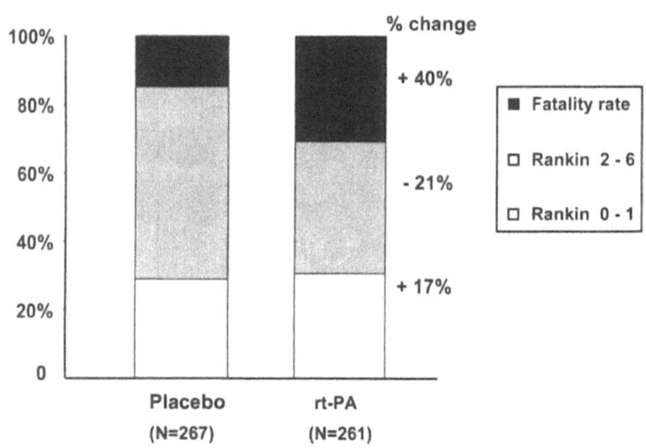

Fig. 3. ECASS trial: Clinical outcome of patients treated after 3 hours

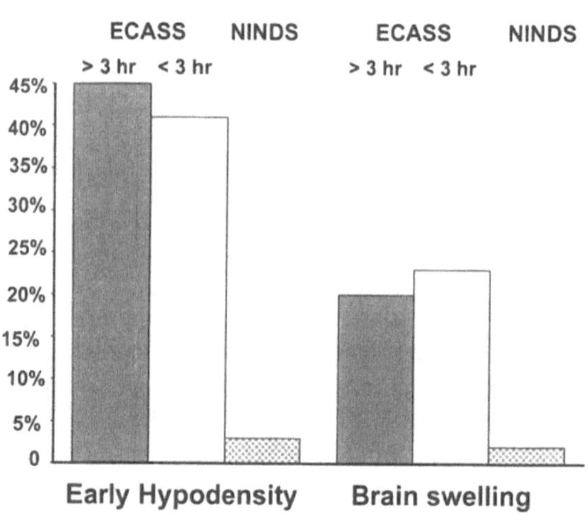

Fig. 4. Early CT signs: ECASS vs NINDS patients

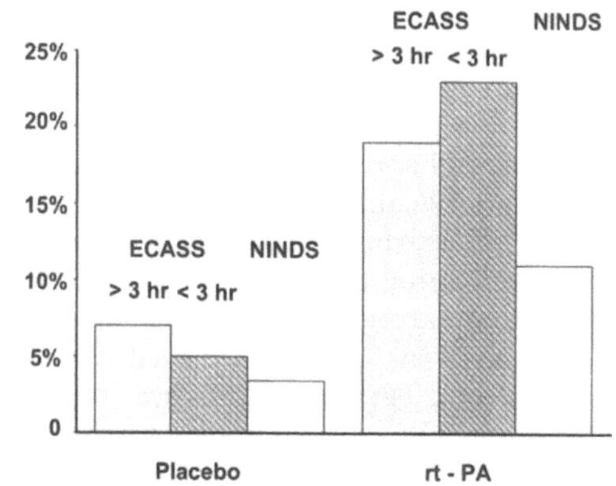

Fig. 5. Parenchymal hemorrhage: ECASS vs NINDS

Interarterial Thrombolytic Therapy for Acute Stroke

Approximately 1200 strokes occur each day in the US. One-third of these patients die, and another one-third will be permanently disabled. Three million people who have survived a stroke are currently living in the United States [7]. Stroke is the third leading cause of death in the US, at a cost of $ 40 billion/year.

The natural history of middle cerebral artery (MCA) occlusion produces 30% immediate mortality, 40%–65% severe long term disability, and only 12.5% minor non-disabling deficits [8]. The natural history of posterior fossa and basilar occlusions is even worse, with immediate mortality near 86%, severe long-term disability at 10%, and minor nondisabling deficits at 4%.

Improving these odds is likely to require both lysing the clot and re-establishing perfusion. Local intra-arterial thrombolytic therapy is a useful approach to these problems.

The most important thrombolysis considerations are the clinical condition of the patient, the extent of thrombus, the presence of collateral circulation, the time of onset, and CT/MRI evidence that the infarction is non-hemorrhagic. We are now trying to treat all anterior circulation strokes within 6 hours from time of onset and all posterior fossa strokes within 12 hours. The approach includes systemic anticoagulation (bolus dose of 5,000 units of heparin for a 70-kg patient), placement of a micro-catheter directly into the thrombus, and doses of urokinase 50.000 units every 10 minutes, with angiography every 30 minutes to document clot lysis. In the anterior circulation 500,000–750,000 units of urokinase is usually used. In the posterior circulation the dose is between 750,000 and 1 million units of urokinase.

New microcatheters and guidewires permit access to all areas of the anterior circulation, including the distal internal carotid artery, the middle cerebral artery, and the M2 and M3 branches, plus the anterior cerebral artery. In the posterior circulation it is possible to catheterize the distal vertebral artery, basilar artery, and both the posterior cerebral arteries (P1 and P2 segments) for clot lysis. Figure 7 is the case of a 51-year-old man who presented with symptoms of a right hemispheric stroke due to right internal carotid artery occlusion. Six months later he presented with a left internal carotid artery occlusion and was very lethargic and hemiparetic on the right side. The left common carotid angiogram showed flow to the external carotid arteries but no filling of the cervical internal carotid artery and poor filling of the supraclinoid carotid artery from external carotid artery collaterals (Fig. 6a). The patient continued to deteriorate despite 2 hours of heparin therapy. A microcatheter was therefore placed from the common carotid up through the cervical internal carotid, through the thrombus into the petrous carotid artery segment (Fig. 6b). After 600,000 units of urokinase, lysis of all of the clot was achieved in the internal carotid artery (Fig. 6c). Angioplasty of a petrous stenosis was then done for complete recanalization. At 6 months of follow-up the patient has done well. Similar good results are possible with middle cerebral artery and basilar artery occlusions.

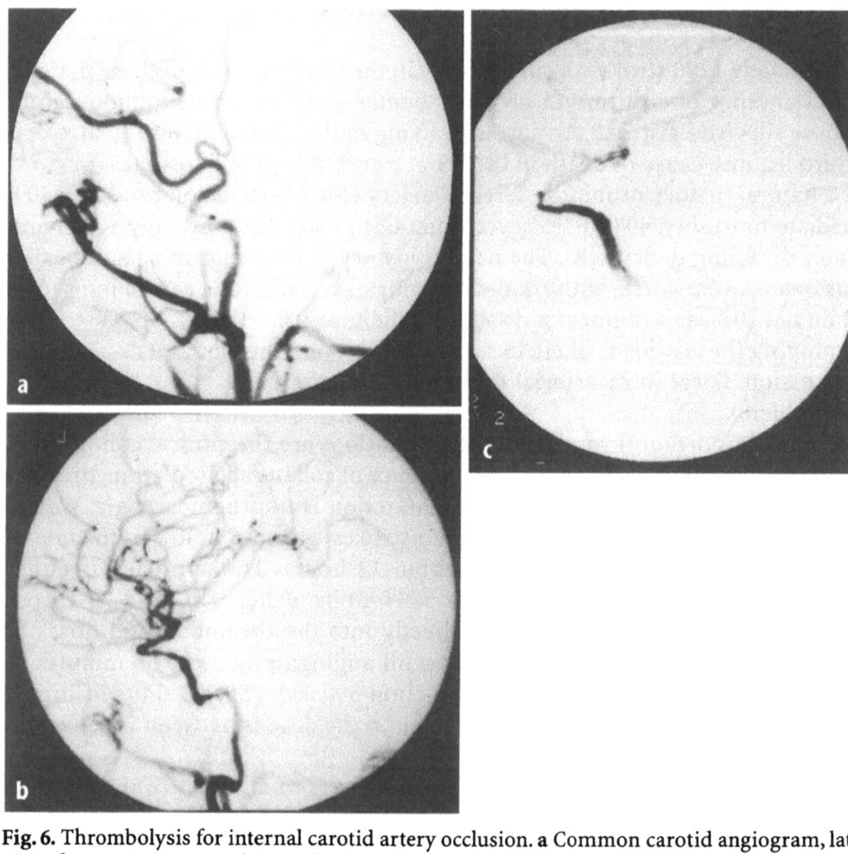

Fig. 6. Thrombolysis for internal carotid artery occlusion. **a** Common carotid angiogram, lateral view, demonstrates complete occlusion of internal carotid artery. **b** Microcatheter placement through the thrombus with infusion of urokinase into the clot. **c** Cleared artery after catheterization and urokinase. Post-treatment after direct urokinase infusion demonstrates reperfusion of intracranial blood vessels

We have treated 27 patients with intra-arterial thrombolysis of this type, in cases involving 45 vascular territories. Treatment produced neurological improvement in 63% of cases (17/27). There were two major strokes (7.4%), and the overall mortality at 6 months of follow-up was 29.6% (8/27).

Hacke and Zeumer et al. reported similar results [9]. In 22 patients with basilar artery occlusions treated only with systemic heparin, the mortality rate was 91%. However, mortality dropped to 65% with intra-arterial urokinase and to 40% with higher doses of either rt-PA or urokinase. Zeumer also reported an 85% recanalization rate in 20 patients with carotid occlusions treated with intra-arterial thrombolytic agents [10].

Tsai also reported intra-arterial thrombolysis in 29 patients with basilar artery occlusions. Mortality was 17%, and survival was 83%, of which 75% had good outcomes [11]. In 33 middle cerebral artery occlusions Tsai et al. reported hemorrhagic transformation in 21% of patients, clinical improvement in 64%, and 6% overall mortality. Mayer et al. reported 49 patients with basilar artery thrombosis treated with intra-arterial lytic agents. Mortality was 47%, and survival was 53%, of which 65% had good outcomes [12]. Brucker et al. reported similar results in 28 cases and observed a high correlation of reperfusion with good clinical outcome [13].

These studies were the basis for the PROACT (Prolyse (recombinant prourokinase) for Acute Cerebral Thromboembolism) Trial. This was a double-blind, prospective, placebo-controlled trial to evaluate recanalization, safety, and clinical outcome of acute embolic strokes in the middle cerebral artery. Treatment was instituted within 6 hours of symptom onset. Investigators screened 1,361 stroke patients, of whom 105 went on to diagnostic arteriography. Forty patients were randomized: 26 to prourokinase and 14 to placebo. Endpoints were recanalization, safety, and clinical outcome.

The angiographic recanalization rate was 56% in the treatment arm vs 15.4% with placebo. With treatment, 36% of recanalizations were complete, vs none with placebo. Treated patients also showed significant improvement on the NIH Stroke Scale, Rankin Scale, and Barthel Index at 90 days after symptom onset. The conclusion was that the recanalization rate with 6 mg of recombinant prourokinase is significantly better than placebo, that safety appears equivalent, and that recanalization appears to correlate with improved stroke outcome at 90 days. This approach will be tested further in Phase 3 studies [14].

Summary: New Aspects of Thrombolysis

A summary of current thinking was presented at the 4th International Symposium on Thrombolytic Therapy in Acute Ischemic Stroke held May 30-Jun 1 in Copenhagen, Denmark. There was no general agreement on the question of whether thrombolysis for acute ischemic stroke should be implemented on the basis of current data.

The risk of death according to clinical state was illustrated with data from the ECASS trial (Fig. 7). Mortality with rt-PA is on the right side of each quadrangle,

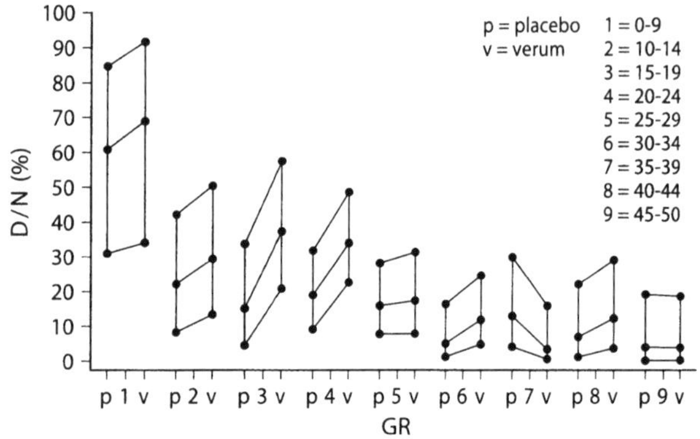

Fig. 7. Risk of death and status on Scandinavian stroke scale

and mortality with placebo is on the left side in this figure. Patients with very severe stroke had mortality of 60–70%, which was higher in the rt-PA group. Mortality was lower in patients with less severe strokes on this univariate analysis.

Multivariate analysis of the ECASS data showed that poor outcome was predicted by age, initial neurological deficit, time to treatment, early extended hypodensity on CT, stroke type, diabetes, and atrial fibrillation. No single factor predicted poor outcome in the NINDS trial, although patients who developed symptomatic hemorrhage had presented with more severe stroke at baseline.

Data from the MAST-Italy trial [15] showed that streptokinase treatment was significantly and independently associated with risk of hemorrhagic transformation and in-hospital death. The MAST-Europe trial [16] found that bad functional outcome was predicted by baseline neurological score and that death at 6 months was predicted by neurological score, age, and streptokinase treatment. The ASK study from Australia [17] concluded that the ability to predict outcome was poor, so there is no consensus on which factors predict poor response to thrombolytic therapy.

Predictors of good outcome include age below 70, rt-PA treatment, no infarction on CT scan, and less severe strokes.

Conclusion

Thrombolysis provides a clear benefit in some patients with acute ischemic stroke. The current problem is that we are not yet able to determine exactly which patients will benefit and when thrombolysis should be used. Optimal therapy is likely to require combination therapy and to be possible only after more is known about the characteristics of clots responsible for the ischemia and about the mechanism responsible for thrombolysis-related hemorrhage.

References

1. Hacke W, Kaste M, Fieschi C, et al (1995) Intravenous thrombolysis with recombinant tissue plasminogen activator for acute hemispheric stroke, The European Cooperative Acute Stroke Study (ECASS). JAMA 274:1017–1025
2. NINDS rt-PA Stroke Study Group (1995) Tissue plasminogen activator for acute ischemic stroke. N Engl J Med 333:1581–1587
3. Brott TG, Haley EC, Levy DE, et al (1992) Urgent therapy for stroke. I. Pilot study of tissue plasminogen activator administered within 90 minutes. Stroke 23:632–640
4. Haley EC Jr, Levy DE, Trott TG, et al (1992) Urgent therapy for stroke. II. Pilot study of tissue plasminogen activator administered 91–180 minutes from onset. Stroke 23:641–645
5. The European Ad Hoc Consensus Group (1996) European strategies for early intervention in stroke. Cerebrovascular Dis 6:315–324
6. Steiner T, Bluhmki E, Kaste M, Toni D, Trouillas P, v. Kummer R, Hacke W, for the ECASS Study Group (1998) The ECASS 3-hour cohort - secondary analysis of ECASS data by time stratification. Cerebrovasc Dis 667 (in press)
7. The National Advisory Neurological Disorders and Stroke Council (1992) Stroke and cererovascular diseases. NIH report, Bethesda, pp 26–27
8. Acheson J, Hutchinson EC (1971) The natural history of focal cerebrovascular disease. Am J Medicine 157:15–25
9. Hacke W, Zeumer H, Ferbert A, et al (1988) Intraarterial thrombolytic therapy improves outcome in patients with acute vertebrobasilar occlusive disease. Stroke 19:1216–1222
10. Zeumer H, Freitag NJ, Knoupe V (1992) Intravascular thrombolysis in central nervous system cerebrovascular disease. Neuroimaging Clinics of North America 2:359–369
11. Tsai FY (1994) Acute thrombolysis of the intracranial dural sinus - direct thrombolytic treatment. Amer J Neurorad 12:1137–1142
12. Meyer H (1994) Proceedings from the ASNR Scientific Meeting, Seattle, May 15–20, 1994
13. Bruckner E (1994) Proceedings from the ASNR Scientific Meeting, Seattle, May 15–20, 1994
14. del Zoppo GJ, Higashida R, Furber TJ, et al (submitted for publication). PROACT: A phase II randomized trial of recombinant pro-urokinase by direct arterial delivery in acute middle cerebral artery thrombosis
15. Multicentre Acute Stroke Trial - Italy (MAST-I) Group (1995) Randomised controlled trial of streptokinase, aspirin, and combination of both in treatment of acute ischaemic stroke. Lancet 346:1509–1514
16. Hommel M, Boissel JP, Cornu C, for the MAST Study Group (1994) Termination of trial of streptokinase in severe acute ischemic stroke. Lancet 345:57
17. Donnan GA, Davis SM, Chambers BR, et al (1994) Letter. Lancet 345:578–579

Preventing Postischemic Injury During Reperfusion

R. C. Koehler, J. R. Kirsch, A. Bhardwaj, H. Takahashi, and R. J. Traystman

Introduction

With the advent of thrombolysis and the ability to reperfuse during focal ischemia, the question arises of what type of neuroprotective drugs can be used in combination with thromblytic therapy to prevent focal injury from occurring. From an experimental point of view, there are three groups: anti-excitatory drugs, antioxidants, and inhibitors of leukocyte inflammatory response.

NMDA Receptor Antagonists

NMDA antagonists are very effective in animal models of focal ischemia but have a rather narrow therapeutic window [1], presumably because the intracellular calcium increase and neuronal depolarization are fairly early events [2, 3]. The NMDA receptor antagonists under study include non-competitive antagonists (phencyclidine, MK-801), competitive antagonists (CPP, CGS19755, NPC17742), glycine site antagonists, polyamine modulatory site, and sigma ligands.

We studied the competitive NMDA antagonist NPC 17742 in a cat model in which the middle cerebral artery was occluded for 60 or 90 minutes (Fig. 1). The drug administration was started 15 minutes before the occlusion was released and reperfusion started. The amount of cortical injury was markedly reduced in treated animals compared to controls with there was a short (60 minute) period of ischemia and the drug was administered at 45 minutes of ischemia, 15 minutes before reperfusion [4]. The degree of protection was markedly diminished if the period of ischemia was extended to 90 minutes and the NMDA antagonists was delayed for only 30 minutes, beginning at 75 minutes of ischemia [5]. This suggests that the efficacy of NMDA antagonists will probably depend on very early administration. Another concern with these drugs is the risk of psychological adverse effects [6].

Another approach to neuroprotection has been inhibition of glutamate release. Drugs under investigation for this purpose include sodium channel inhibitors (lamotrigine, BW 1003C87, BW619C89, lubezole), N-type calcium channel inhibitors, adenosine receptor agonists, and sigma ligands.

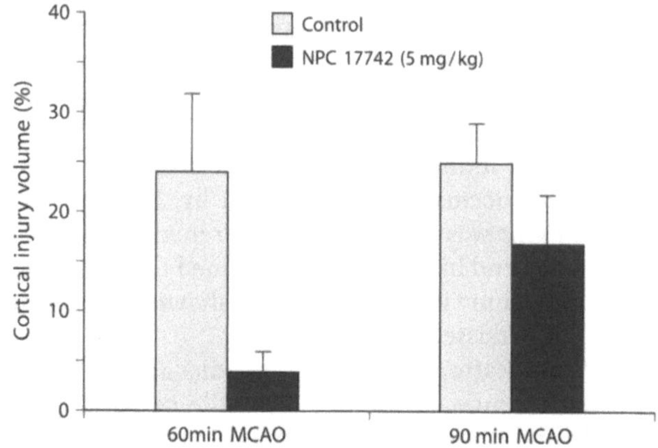

Fig. 1. Effect of competitive NMDA antagonist after middle cerebral artery occlusion in the cat

Sigma Ligands

Sigma ligand receptors appear in both of these neuroprotector categories. These receptors are now beginning to be described molecularly [7], so information about them is based on pharmacological evidence. They are non-opioid ligand binding sites in specific regions throughout the central nervous system (CNS). They are not blocked by naloxone. Sigma-1 receptors are thought to be linked to G-proteins. Sigma receptors interact with various transmitter systems in different regions of the CNS. They inhibit glutamate release in glutaminergic neurons, norepinephrine uptake in catecholaminergic neurons in the striatum that can modulate dopamine release, and affect acetylcholine release. They have different functions in different parts of the brain [8]. There is some evidence in tissue culture that sigma ligands can prevent excitotoxic injury [9]. There is also work in the gerbil showing that sigma ligands can provide neuroprotection in global ischemia [10–13]. We thought it would be useful to look at these ligands to see if they can decrease injury in focal ischemia.

The hypothesis tested was that IV administration of a potent sigma-receptor ligand during transient focal ischemia could decrease brain injury. The first ligand studied was PPBP (4-phenyl-1-(4-phenylbutyl) piperidine.) Two injury models were used. An acute model in cats was used to measure cerebral blood flow and determine whether the drug is reducing injury by improving CBF or by providing direct neuroprotection [14]. This model included 90 minutes of middle cerebral artery occlusion and 240 minutes of reperfusion. PPBP was given at 0.1 umol/kg/hr or at 1.0 umol/kg/hr beginning at 75 minutes of occlusion and continuing throughout the reperfusion period.

The higher dose of PPBP significantly reduced the injury volume, expressed as a percent of total caudate or cortex volume (Fig. 2). Examination of 12 coronal sections showed that the injury was reduced at all levels (Fig. 3).

A microsphere technique was used to measure cerebral blood flow (CBF). This showed that there was neuroprotection in the low-dose group even though CBF remained markedly reduced. Technical problems interfered with interpretation of CBF results in the high-dose animals.

The other model was in the rat, in which 120 minutes of suture middle cerebral artery occlusion was followed by 22 hours of reperfusion [15]. PPBP at 1 umol/kg/hr was given throughout reperfusion. The experiment was carried out for one day and histology was examined the following day. There was a reduction in injury volume in the treated rats, showing that protection was not just an acute effect but persisted at 24 hours.

The implication of these two studies is that the sigma-receptor ligand PPBP decreases injury volume from middle cerebral artery occlusion in cat and rat models, and that the mechanism is not secondary to a more favorable redistribution of cerebral blood flow.

The second drug studied was pentazocine [16], which was developed many years ago for psychiatric use. The positive isomer of pentazocine has very high selectivity and specificity as a sigma-1 ligand. The negative isomer is a non-specific opioid ligand and probably causes some of the psychosis and hallucinations that occur with high doses of racemic pentazocine. We compared the effects of the two isomers in the rat model, which included 2 hours of ischemia and 22 hours of reperfusion, with the drug given at 2 mg/kg/hr as a continuous infusion beginning after 1 hour of ischemia. Infarct volume was measured at 24 hours.

The positive isomer of pentazocine significantly reduced the infarct volume both in the cortex and in the striatum (Fig. 4). Animals who received the negative isomer had infarct volumes similar to those of untreated controls. The results with the positive isomer in the striatum are particularly promising because the striatum is end-artery region in which it is often very difficult to provide neuroprotection.

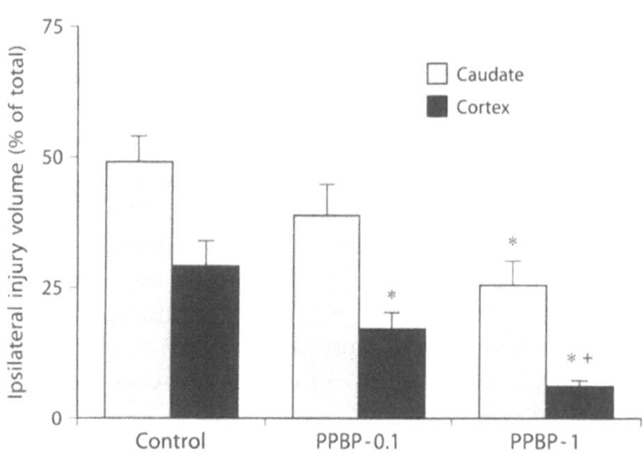

Fig. 2. PPBP reduces injury volume in cat acute ischemia model – * $P < 0.05$ from control group; + $P < 0.05$ between 0.1 and 1.0 umol/kg/hr infusion doses of PPBP, reprinted from Takahashi [14]

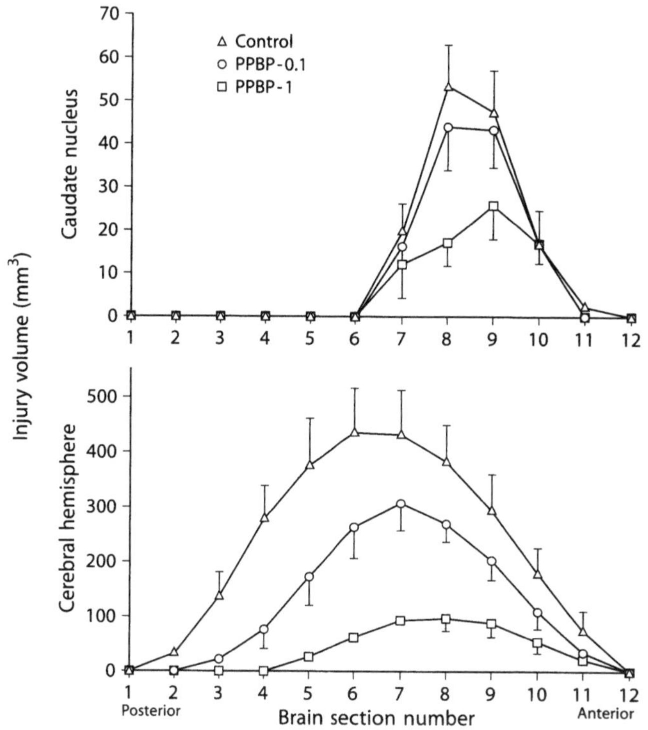

Fig. 3. PPBP reduced injury at all coronal levels in cat acute ischemia model, reprinted from Takahashi [14]

These studies indicate that sigma receptors are important in the mechanism of injury following middle cerebral artery occlusion and that they may be important targets for pharmacologic manipulation. The mechanism of this effect may involve modulation of NMDA receptor function. One way NMDA receptors seem to be involved in injury is via nitric oxide synthase, at least in cell cultures [17]. With injury-related calcium influx there is overstimulation of the calcium-dependent enzyme, resulting in overproduction of nitric oxide. This combines with superoxide to generate toxic peroxynitrite and hydroxyl radicals.

Nitric oxide (NO) was examined by Bhardwaj et al. using in vivo microdialysis [18]. This method uses a microdialysis probe into the striatum perfused with radio-labeled arginine, while measuring radiolabeled citrulline in the effluent. For every mole of NO produced, one mole of arginine is converted to one mole of citrulline. The citrulline level increased markedly following middle cerebral artery occlusion but not in animals who had sham neck surgery. We believe this reflects an increase in nitric oxide production in this model of focal ischemia.

This model was then used to examine the effects of various agents. When one millimolar NMDA was perfused through the microdialysis probe, the citrulline

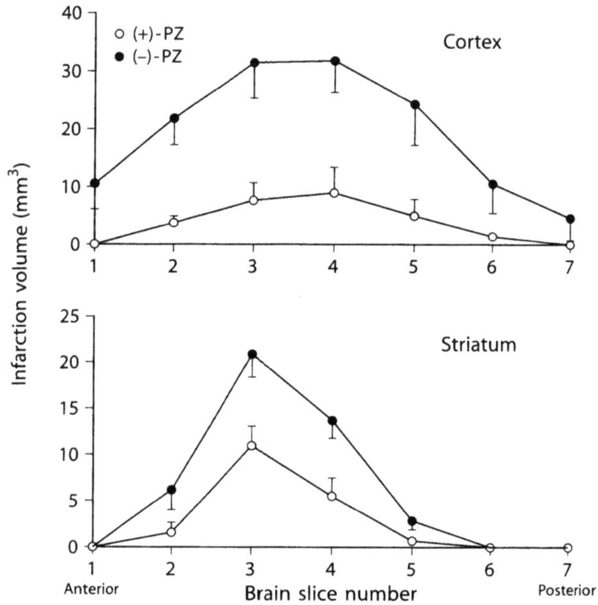

Fig. 4. Effect of positive vs negative pentazocine isomers on infarction volume

recovery increased. This indicates that NMDA is capable of increasing the turnover of arginine and hence presumably NO production in vivo in the striatum. When the positive isomer of pentazocine was given together with NMDA, the citrulline recovery was reduced. We posulate that pentazocine could be modifying NMDA function in such as way as to reduce the overproduction of nitric oxide.

Conclusion

Our conclusion is that sigma ligands are capable of inhibiting NMDA-invoked increases in nitric oxide production and that they are neuroprotective, not only in global ischemia but also in focal ischemia. One way to tailor neuropharmacology in the future may be to modulate specific effects rather than just completely inhibiting NMDA receptors. There may be ways to pharmacologically design sigma ligands specific for the sigma-1 receptor that would not have the adverse effects of some other neuroprotective drugs.

References

1. Margaill I, Parmentier S, Callebert J, et al (1996) Short therapeutic window for MK-801 in transient focal cerebral ischemia in mornotensive rats. J Cereb Blood Flow Metab 16: 107–113
2. DeGraba TJ, Ostrow PT, Grotta JC (1993) Threshold of calcium disturbances after focal cerebral ischemia in rats. Stroke 24: 1212–1217
3. Gill R, Andine P, Hillered L, et al (1992) The effect of MK-801 on cortical spreading depression in the penumbral zone following focal ischemia in the rat. J Cereb Blood Flow Metab 12:371–379
4. Nishikawa T, Kirsch JR, Koehler RC, et al (1994) Competitive N-methyl-D-aspartate receptor blockage reduces brain injury following transient focal ischemia in cats. Stroke 25: 2258–2264
5. Miyabe M, Kirsch JR, Nishikawa T, et al (1997) Comparative analysis of brain protection by N-methyl-D-aspartate receptor antagonists after transient focal ischemia in cats. Crit Care Med 25: 1037–1043
6. Muir KW, Lees KR (1995) Clinical experience with excitatory amino acid antagonist drugs. Stroke 26: 503–513
7. Hanner M, Moebius FF, Flandorfer A, et al (1996) Purification, molecular cloning, and expression of the mammalian sigma-binding site. Proc Natl Aca Sci USA 93: 8072–8077
8. Walker JM, Bowen WD, Walker FO, et al (1990) Sigma receptors: biology and function. Pharmacol Rev 42: 355–402
9. Lockhart BP, Soulard P, Benicourt C, et al (1995) Distinct neuroprotective profiles for sigma ligands against N-methyl-D-aspartate (NMDA), and hypoxia-mediated neurotoxicity in neuronal culture toxicity studies. Brain Res 675: 110–120
10. Lysko PG, Feuerstein G (1990) Excitatory amino acid neurotoxicity at the N-methyl-D-aspartate receptor in cultured neurons: protection by SKF 10,047. Neurosci Lett 120: 217–220
11. Contreras PC, Gray NM, Ragan DM, et al (1992) BMY-14802 protects against ischemia-induced neuronal damage in the gerbil. Life Sci 51: 1145–1149
12. Lysko PG, Yue T-L, Gu J-L, et al (1992) Neuroprotective mechanism of (+) SKF 10,047 in vitro and in gerbil global brain ischemia. Stroke 23: 1319–1324
13. O'Neill M, Caldwell M, Earley B, et al (1995) The sigma receptor ligand JO 1784 (igmesine hydrochloride) is neuroprotective in the gerbil model of global cerebral ischemia. Eur J Pharmacol 283: 217–225
14. Takahashi H, Kirsch JR, Hashimoto K, et al (1995) PPBP [4-phenyl-1-(4-phenylbutyl) piperidine], a potent sigma-receptor ligand, decreases brain injury following transient focal ischemia in cats. Stroke 26: 1676–1682
15. Takahashi H, Kirsch JR, Hashimoto K, et al (1996) PPBP [4-phenyl-1-(4-phenylbutyl) piperidine] decreases brain injury after transient focal ischemia in rats. Stroke 27: 2120–2123
16. Takahashi H, Traystman RJ, Hashimoto K, et al (1997) Postischemic brain injury is affected stereospecifically by pentazocine in rats. Anesth Analg 85: 353–357
17. Lesage AS, De Loore KL, Peeters L, et al (1995) Neuroprotective sigma ligands interefere with the glutamate-activated NOS pathway in hippocampal cell culture. Synapse 20: 156–164
18. Bhardwaj A, Northington FJ, Hanley DF, et al (1996) Striatal nitric oxide (NO) production is enhanced in focal cerebral ischemia: An in vivo microdialysis study. Presented at a meeting on Emergency Management and Critical Care of Stroke, Heidelberg, September 1996

Mechanisms of Reversible Injury and Neuroprotection

R. J. Traystman and M. Hennerici

Introduction

A key element of the emerging strategy for acute care of stroke is to protect brain tissue from damage until cerebral blood flow can be restored. To that end a number of potential neuroprotective drugs are now in clinical trials.

Neuroprotection: From Basic Science to Phase II

There are at least three mechanisms by which ischemia can produce neuronal death or injury: free radicals, excitotoxicity, and inflammatory mediators. Free radicals formed following an ischemic event can cause cell membrane destruction and neuronal death. Ischemia causes the release of a variety of excitotoxic amino acids such as glutamate and aspartate. These affect various receptor sites, including the NMDA site which mediates calcium fluxes, and the quisqualate and kainate receptors which mediate sodium and chloride fluxes. When activated, these receptors cause the opening of channels and changes in intracellular ion concentrations, eventually leading to cell death. Mediators of inflammation such as leukotrienes and platelet activating factors can similarly cause membrane damage and cell death. Many treatment modalities have been used in attempts to protect the brain. These include:
- Hypothermia
- Barbiturates
- Free radical scavengers
- Excitatory amino acid blockers
- Calcium channel blockers
- Heparin
- Nitric oxide synthase inhibitors
- Tissue plasminogen activator

Early preclinical work with drugs such as MK801, both pre-ischemia and post-ischemia, illustrates the research problems we face in trying to match up animal studies with clinical drug development for stroke victims [1]. MK801 can reduce infarct volume by 40–50% and is effective even if given after ischemia is induced. MK801 is unlikely to have clinical application because of human toxicity problems, but it does indicate that research with excitatory amino acid antagonists should be pursued. Other agents, including the MK801-like agent (2R,4R,5S-[2-amino-4,5-1,2-cyclohexyl-7-phosphonoheptanoic acid]) (NPC 17742), can reduce infarct volume by about 50% and are effective not only in the caudate but also in the cerebral hemispheres [2].

Free radical scavengers such as polyethylene glycol-conjugated superoxide dismutase (PEG-SOD) can also reduce infarct volume by about 50% [3]. A similar reduction in infarct size occurs with L-NAME, a nitric oxide synthase inhibitor, given either pre-ischemia or post-ischemia. L-NAME is effective in the caudate but less so in the cerebral hemispheres [4].

Considerable preclinical work has been done using middle cerebral artery (MCA) occlusion models, but these studies are not easily comparable. Problems include differences in variables measured, such as cerebral blood flow, arterial pressure, duration of the occlusion, and drug doses. Often the test drugs are given only at a single dose level, not at high, middle, and low doses to permit dose-response examination of putative drug-specific effects.

The timing of drug administration is also important. Is it given at reperfusion or 15 minutes, 30 minutes, 1 hour or 6 hours after the reperfusion has begun? The animal species used is also important. Different species sometimes give different results. Almost everything works in the gerbil model, but almost nothing works in the cat, dog, monkey, or human. Different surgical techniques may also influence outcome. The use of string versus neurosurgical vascular clips may affect the results. Finally, the choice of anesthetic is important. Different anesthetics have different effects on the cerebral circulation and cerebral function.

The process of preclinical development can be illustrated by work done on the amino steroid tirilazad. This drug has a vitamin E-like scavenging effect on lipid peroxide radicals. It scavenges oxygen radicals, particularly superoxide, and stabilizes membranes.

We studied tirilazad in a global ischemia model in which we could control cerebral perfusion pressure to a level of ischemia of about 10 mmHg. Tirilazad was compared to placebo in a randomized, blinded study [5]. NMR spectrometer data showed that the brain intracellular pH and bicarbonate fall markedly with either drug or placebo but return toward normal faster with tirilazad than with vehicle (Fig. 1). Similarly, somatosensory evoked potentials fall to zero during ischemia but return to about 40–50 % with tirilazad during reperfusion, versus 20–30% with vehicle.

In a more severe model which produces hyperglycemia in addition to ischemia, evoked potentials did not return from zero after reperfusion in control animals but returned to about 40% of baseline after 3 hours of reperfusion in tirilazad-treated animals. Intracellular pH and bicarbonate similarly do not recover very much in control animals but return to about 70% of baseline in tirilazad-treated animals (Fig. 2).

Dose-response curves are important and often neglected in preclinical studies of neuroprotective drugs. These can be examined not only for pH but also for high-energy phosphates. In the animal model, phosphocreatine and ATP recovered after reperfusion in a dose-dependent fashion in animals treated with tirilazad (Fig. 3).

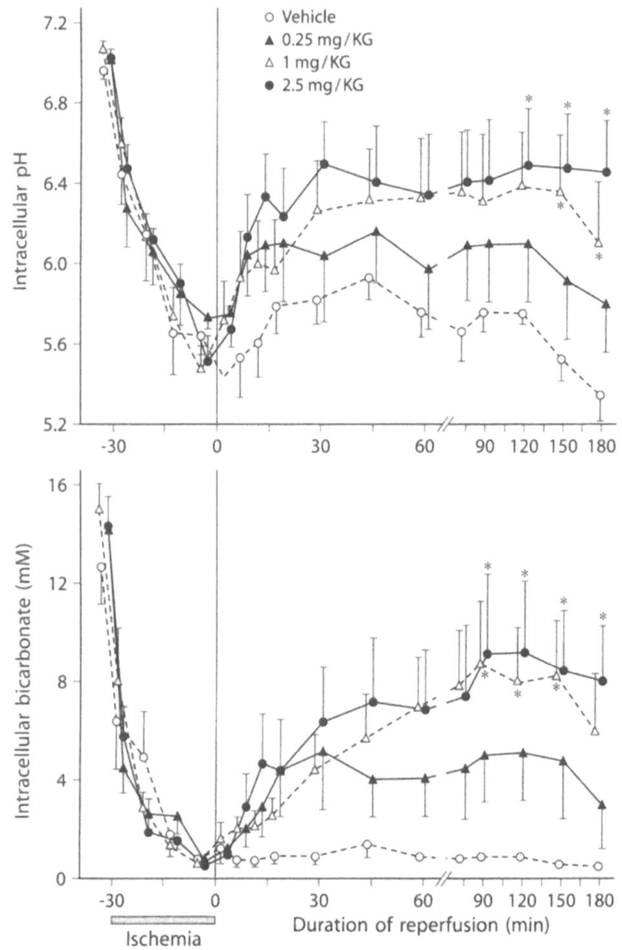

Fig. 1. Effect of tirilazad on intracellular pH in ischemia; line graphs show intracellular pH and calculated intracellular bicarbonate ion concentration during and after 30 min of hyperglycemic, incomplete ischemia in dogs treated with vehicle or 0.25, 1.0, or 2.5 mg/kg of tirilazad at reperfusion. Bars represent SME. Zero time indicates start of reperfusion. Time scale is compressed after 60 min to highlight early transients. * $P < 0.05$ from vehicle group. From: Kim H, et al (1996) Stroke 27:114–121

Finally, it will be increasingly important to consider combinations of drugs in preclinical studies. As discussed in Chapter 11 by Drs. Zivin and Grotta, the selection of combinations will be most likely based upon the different mechanisms of action of these drugs. For example, we have used deferoxamine, an oxygen radical scavenger, combined with GPI, which is an excitatory amino acid blocker. We found that cerebral blood flow is similar with these drugs under normal circumstances and during ischemia. However, during reperfusion the highest cerebral blood flow was obtained with the combined drugs (Fig. 4). The highest level of

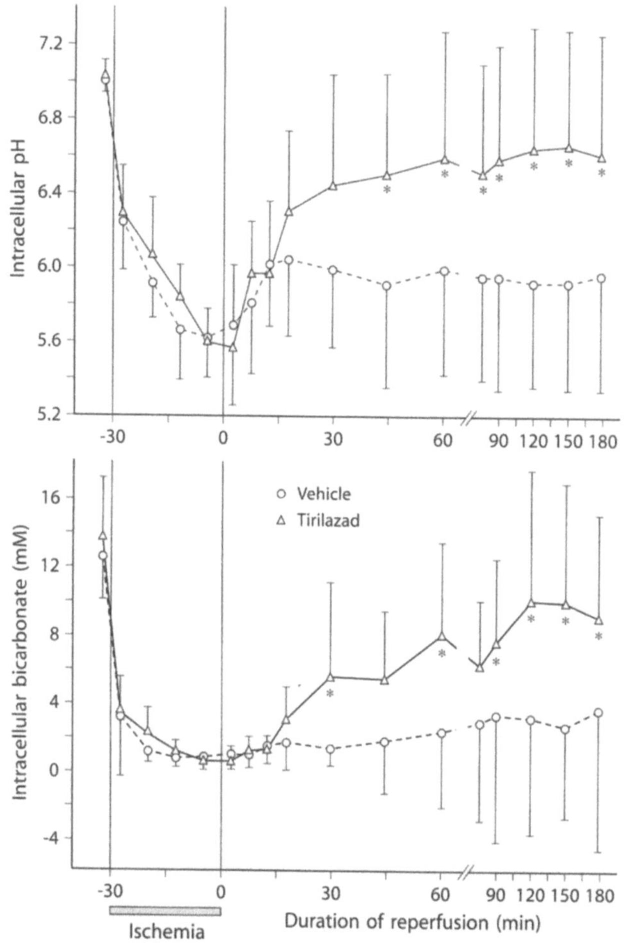

Fig. 2. Effect of tirilazad on intracellular pH in more severe hyperglycemic incomplete ischemia; intracellular pH (top) and intracellular bicarbonate ion concentration (bottom) estimated from intracellular pH and sagittal sinus PCO_2 during 30 min of hyperglycemic ischemia and 180 min of reperfusion in dogs pretreated with vehicle (n=8) or tirilazad (n=8). Zero time indicates start of reperfusion. Time is compressed after 60 min to highlight early transients. * $P<0.05$ between groups by two-way analysis of variance and orthogonal contrasts. Values are means ± SD. From: Maruki Y, et al (1995) J Cereb Blood Flow & Metab 15:88–96

intracellular pH following reperfusion was also in the animals who received both drugs (Fig. 5). Phosphocreatine and ATP levels also returned significantly more toward baseline in animals who received both drugs (Fig. 6).

Major problems still must be overcome to achieve adequate neuroprotection. The first is getting the patient to the hospital more quickly after the stroke occurs. A second is determining the window of opportunity for these drugs: When do potential neuroprotective agents have to be given? The next problem is drug

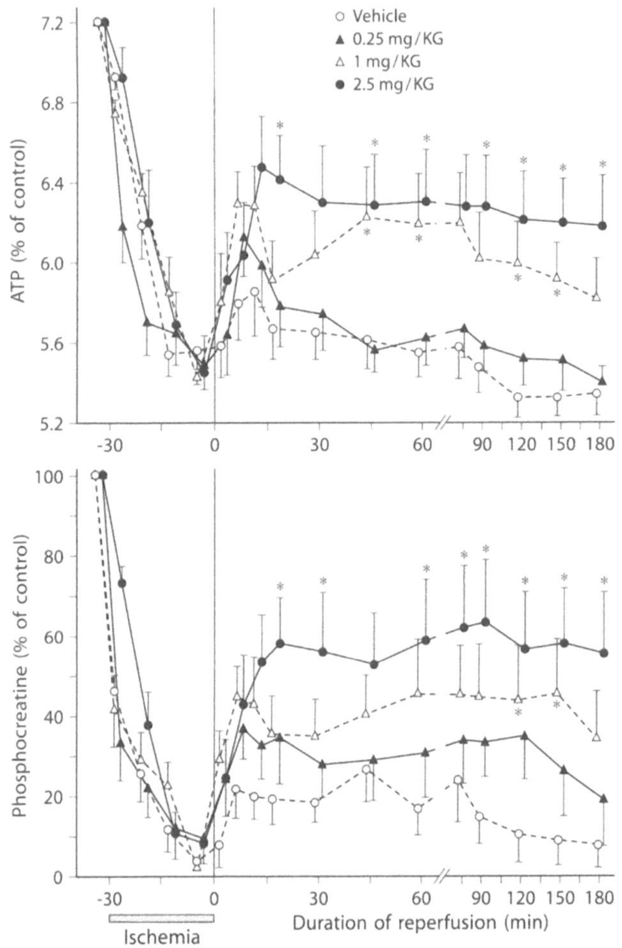

Fig. 3. Dose-dependent recovery of phosphocreatine with tirilazad treatment at reperfusion. Line graphs show cerebral ATP and phosphocreatine during and after 30 min of hyperglycemic, incomplete ischemia in dogs treated with vehicle or 0.25, 1.0, or 2.5 mg/kg of tirilazad at reperfusion. Bars represent SEM. Zero time indicates start of reperfusion. Time scale is compressed after 60 minutes to highlight early transients. * $P < 0.05$ from vehicle group. From: Kim H, et al (1996) Stroke 27:114–121

dose. Some drugs work well at low doses but not at high doses. Others work at high but not low doses. Yet other drugs work well in the middle range but not at the extremes. Full dose-response curves will be needed to determine optimal drug dose. The final issue is how to choose the best combination of drugs for the "cocktail" approach. This will require thinking mechanistically about what we are trying to block to effectively ameliorate the effects of ischemic damage.

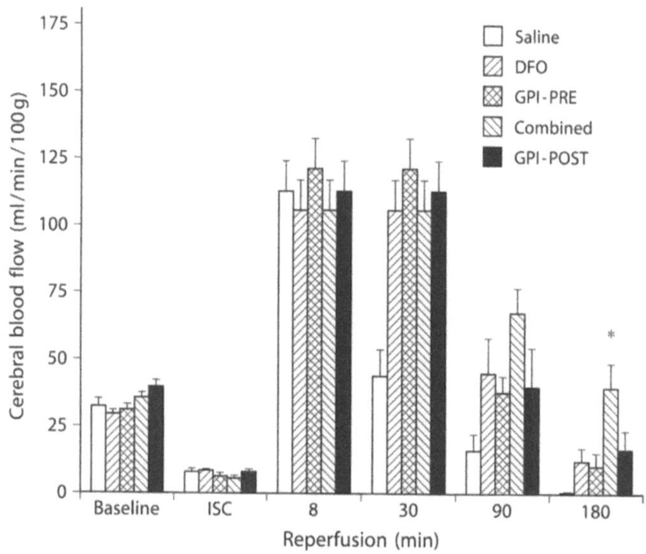

Fig. 4. Effect of combined deferoxamine/GPI on reperfusion CBF. CBF during ischemia and reperfusion. Values (mean ± SD) are shown at baseline, the midpoint of ischemia (ISC) (18 minutes), at four reperfusion time points; n = 8 for all groups. * $P < 0.05$, combined greater than all other groups. From: Davis S, et al (1997) Stroke 28: 198–205

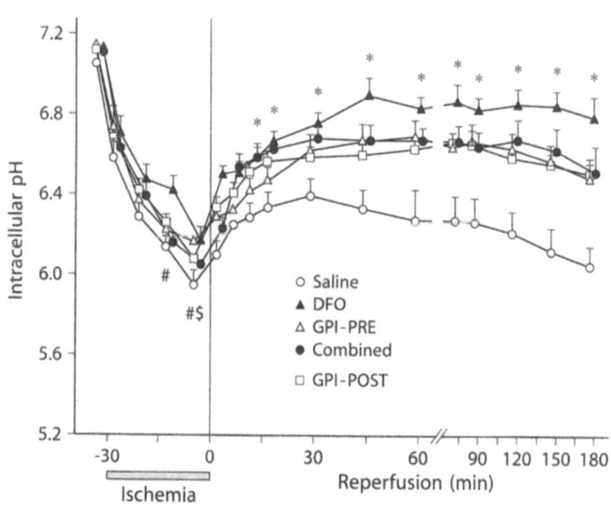

Fig. 5. Effect of Combined Deferoxamine/GPI on Reperfusion Intracellular pH. pH, as determined by 31P MRS and estimated [HCO_3^-] levels during ischemia and reperfusion (mean ± SEM). Zero time indicates the start of reperfusion. Time scale is compressed after 60 min to emphasize early transients; n = 8 for all groups. * $P < 0.05$ compared with saline group; # $P < 0.05$, combined greater than saline; $P < 0.05$, GPI-pre greater than saline. From: Davis S, et al (1997) Stroke 28: 198–205

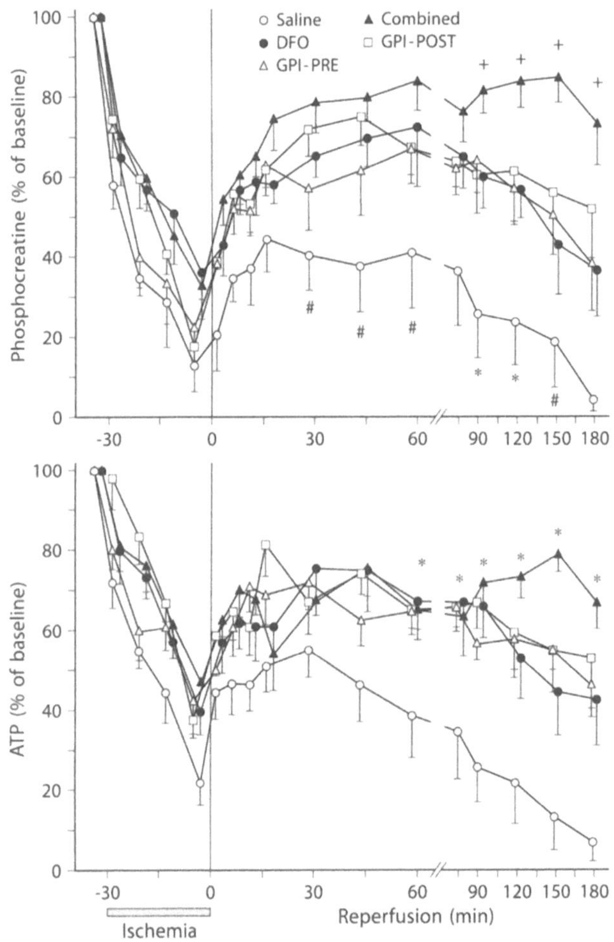

Fig. 6. Effect of combined deferoxamine/GPI on phosphocreatine recovery. Energy phosphate recovery (phosphocreatine and ATP) as determined by 31P MRS (mean ± SEM). Zero time indicates the start of reperfusion. Time scale is compressed after 60 min to emphasize early transients; n = 8 for all groups. * $P < 0.05$., all groups greater than saline; + $P < 0.05$, combined greater than all other groups; # $P < 0.05$, combined greater than saline. From: Davis S, et al (1997) Stroke 28:198–205

Ongoing Human Trials and New Drugs in Acute Stroke

The current situation with neuroprotectants in humans is that virtually nothing has worked so far, but many basic scientific leads are being followed in current clinical trials. Two aspects of the injury mechanism underlying ischemic damage are likely to be important in further developments. The first involves energy. ATP is the major energy reserve in the cell. The mitochondria provide ATP that fuels a multitude of ion pumps which produce and maintain voltage and ion gradients across neurons. The gradients are mostly needed in order to keep high levels of calcium out of the cell or to store it in particular areas, such as the endoplasmic reticulum. In the case of ischemia, energy fails and ATP reduction begins within minutes, causing the calcium influence of this system to fail. The mechanism is generally thought of as excitotoxicity. It assumes that the decrease of membrane potential and the increased release of glutamate all contribute to the increase of intracellular calcium. This cascade, via enzymes and free radicals, is also a pathway leading to apoptosis.

Because calcium plays a major role in this process, clinical trials have investigated whether administration of a calcium antagonist would be useful in reducing morbidity and mortality in acute stroke. A summary of these studies, which have included about 1800 patients, found no benefit for nimodipine versus placebo. Subclass analysis suggested that earlier treatment (i.e. in the first 12 hours after stroke) favored better results, and this should be investigated further.

This again raises the question of whether it is wise to wait to administer neuroprotective drugs until symptoms appear and the patient is at the hospital, or whether another, more modern concept can be developed. For instance, patients who are already at risk because of repeated transient ischemic attacks and the presence of carotid stenosis but who could not undergo surgery could be included in a neuroprotection trial even before they present with symptoms. Thus, they could be prepared to treat themselves early.

Among the more recent neuroprotective drugs in clinical trials are cerestat, lubeluzole, selfotel, clomethiazole, eliprodil, and anti-ICAM-1. Cerestat is a NMDA ion-channel antagonist. A dose-ranging study of 30, 70, and 100 microgram doses has been done. A larger 900-patient study is ongoing in North American and Australia.

Another interesting drug is lubeluzole, a glutamate release antagonist [6]. Whether this is the drug's only or even main action is unknown. Experimental evidence suggests that many of these drugs have two mechanisms of action which are sometimes quite obscure. Animal studies of lubeluzole showed that the drug has a protective effect on neurological function if given at high doses even within 6 hours after onset [7]. With lower doses this effect was smaller and lasted less than 6 hours.

This work led to a series of Phase II and Phase III trials. In the target population lubeluzole at 20 mg/day produced a decrease in the percentage of patients with good functional outcomes and an increase in mortality compared to placebo. Lubeluzole at 10 mg/day, by contrast, both improved outcomes and decreased mortality [8]. In patients with more severe deficits there were similar results.

Two large lubeluzole studies have been completed. These are the European/ Australian Trial (LUB-INT 5) and the North American Trial (LUB-INT 9) [9, 10]. These randomized, multi-center, double-blind, placebo-controlled studies compared lubeluzole at 10 mg/day to placebo, with 361 patients per treatment group.

Eliprodil is a NMDA-polyamine antagonist that is also being studied for neuroprotection. The European sections of the trial were stopped because the statistical board recommended to the steering committee that there would be no benefit demonstrable in the study. The American parts of the trial are still ongoing. The interesting geographic effect may have to do with the use of low-dose heparin rather than with eliprodil itself.

Tirilazad mesylate is a lipid peroxyl radical scavenger. Experimental data from a small study (TESS-1) showed no effect in 414 patients. A new trial of tirilazad at 10 mg/kg is ongoing (TESS-2). Findings in other preliminary human studies of subarachnoid hemorrhage suggested that a higher dose seems indicated in treatment of vasospasm.

Another mechanism that relates to the pathogenesis of a focal ischemic lesion involves the endothelial-leukocyte interaction. The ICAM-1 adhesion molecule appears on vascular endothelium at 1 to 2 hours after onset of ischemia and peaks between 6 and 12 hours. Anti-ICAM-1 is a murine monoclonal antibody which inhibits neutrophil adhesion and migration. It was studied in a European trial which was stopped in 1996 showing no benefit.

Conclusion

Once safety considerations are satisfied, the key questions are those of:

- Efficacy: Does the drug work in ideal conditions?
- Effectiveness: Does the drug work in routine conditions?
- Efficiency: Is there a positive cost/benefit ratio?

All of these trials of potential new neuroprotective agents raise questions about trial design, particular study entry criteria and endpoints. Mortality is important because, as the lubeluzole trial has shown, these drugs can increase mortality by side effect. Morbidity is the most important endpoint, but the question of whether function is the only endpoint is really the most important one. The correlation between clinical criteria and those from experimental studies is also important, measuring infarction volume on one side and an arbitrary functional scales endpoint on the other. Exclusion of patients who are unlikely to benefit, such as those who are comatose or stuporous, is somewhat arbitrary although useful for the sake of the trial. However, at some point we must investigate those patients, because certainly these are patients who could also benefit.

Trials must be designed to minimize the risk of side effects. Cardiovascular, psychomimetic, and neuronal toxic effects can be quite severe and may impede adequate blinding unless the trial is carefully designed.

References

1. Pan Y, Lo EH, Matsumoto K, et al (1995) Quantitative and dynamic MRI of neuroprotection in experimental stroke. J Neurological Sciences 131(2):128–134
2. Nishikawa T, Kirsch JR, Koehler RC, et al (1994) Competitive N-methyl-D-aspartate receptor blockade reduces brain injury following transient focal ischemia in cats. Stroke 25: 2258–2264

3. Matsumiya N, Koehler RC, Kirsch JR, et al (1991) Conjugated superoxide dismutase reduces extent of caudate injury after transient focal ischemia in cats. Stroke 22:1193–1200
4. Nishikawa T, Kirsch JR, Koehler RC, et al (1994) Nitric oxide synthase inhibition reduces caudate injury following transient focal ischemia in cats. Stroke 25:877–885
5. Maruki Y, Koehler RC, Kirsch JR, et al (1995) Tirilazad pretreatment improves early cerebral metabolic and blood flow recovery from hyperglycemic ischemia. J Cerebral Blood Flow & Metabolism 15(1):88–96
6. Haseldonckx M, Van Reempts J, Van de Ven M, et al (1997) Protection with lubeluzole against delayed ischemic brain damage in rats. A quantitative histopathologic study. Stroke 28(2): 428–432
7. De Ryck M, Keersmaekers R, Duytschaever H, et al (1996) Lubeluzole protects sensorimotor function and reduces infarct size in a photochemical stroke model in rats. Journal of Pharmacology & Experimental Therapeutics 279:748–758
8. Diener HC, Hacke W, Hennerici M, et al (1996) Lubeluzole in acute ischemic stroke. A double-blind, placebo-controlled phase II trial. Lubeluzole International Study Group. Stroke 27:76-81
9. European/Australian Lubeluzole Study
10. North American Lubeluzole Study

Combined Neuroprotection/Thrombolysis in Acute Stroke

J. Zivin and J. Grotta

Introduction

The major barrier to effective use of thrombolytic therapy in acute stroke remains the fact that most patients have irreversible damage before it is possible to treat them with these new agents. As discussed elsewhere in this volume, major efforts are being made to bring patients in for treatment earlier in the stroke process. Another approach is to find ways to protect vulnerable brain tissue from ischemic damage long enough to permit the use of thrombolytic therapy.

Multimodal Treatment in Acute Stroke

J. Zivin

As a result of experience with recombinant human tissue plasminogen activator, many investigators no longer believe that placebo-controlled trials in patients treated within 3 hours of symptom onset are justified. Future trials in that time range will thus be combination studies. This increases the importance of effective preclinical evaluation of combination regimens.

Studies of recombinant human tissue plasminogen activator (rt-PA) in combination with other drugs typically use rabbits as the animal model. An important consideration for this animal model is that human rt-PA is about two thirds as effective at dissolving rabbit clots as is native rabbit rt-PA. When differences in kinetics and volume of distribution are taken into account, about twice as much human as rabbit rt-PA is needed to dissolve clots. This is much better than rat models, for example, in which human rt-PA is only about 10% effective for rat clot dissolution. We believe that the large amounts needed in the rat model could affect the kinetics and cause side effects.

The rabbit model involves a simple cutdown in the neck, occlusion of the external carotid artery, and implanting a cannula in the common carotid artery to inject particles. After the surgery is complete, the animal is awake and unanesthetized, so many aspects of physiology which might influence neuroprotection, such as blood pressure, body temperature, and blood gases, are under normal physiologic regulation.

To study ischemic stroke, blood is taken from a donor animal, allowed to form clots, and injected into the carotid circulation. This produces clots in end vessels in the brain. Tracer amounts of radioactive microspheres are injected with the clots and used to measure the specific activity of the brain and to determine how many clots lodge in the brain. The result is small infarcts in random locations throughout the brain.

Data are analyzed by plotting the weight of microspheres, which is a measure of the amount of clot in the brain, versus percent of animals displaying neurologic deficits (Fig. 1). There are two parameters of interest in this curve. One is the position paremeter, which is the mean weight of clots the animal can tolerate. The other is the slope parameter, which is an estimate of the population variance. If the curve shifts to the right it implies that the animals can tolerate more clots. A change in the slope of the curve means that something else has happened. Shifts in the slope typically occur when two effects are taking place at the same time. For example, a drug might provide neuroprotection but simultaneously alters blood pressure. One problem with this model is that there is a ceiling effect. Animals given high doses of clots often die before they can be treated.

Figure 1 illustrates the effect of rt-PA alone in this model [1]. Curve A is the control and shows that the untreated animals tolerated about 3 mg of clots. Curves B, C, and D are the results of treating with rt-PA at 15, 45, and 30 minutes after clots were injected. They show that the treated animals tolerated about three times more clots than the control animals. However, if treatment was delayed for one hour, the curve was not significantly different from the control curve. This was the first demonstration in a clinically applicable model that rt-PA reduced neurologic damage.

This model was used in a study of rtPA and MK-801, which is a glutamate antagonist. MK-801 was given at 1 mg/kg 5 minutes after embolization. rtPA was given at 1 mg/kg at various later times. MK-801 alone had no significant effect. rtPA alone at 60 minutes after embolization nearly doubled the amount of clots the animal could tolerate (Table 1) [2]. Giving both drugs at 60 minutes was more effective than rtPA alone, even though MK-801 was ineffective alone. Delaying rtPA treatment to 90 minutes did not produce a therapeutic effect.

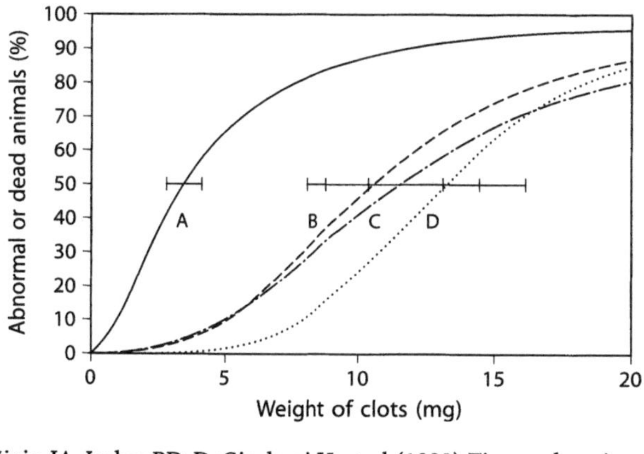

Fig. 1. Effect of rht-PA. (From: Zivin JA, Lyden PD, DeGirolami U, et al (1988) Tissue plasminogen activator. Reduction of neurologic damage after experimental embolic stroke. Arch Neurol 45:387–391)

Table 1. Effects of t-PA and MK-801 on neurologic function. (From [2])

Drug	Dose (mg/kg)	t-PA treatment (min)	$ES_{50} \pm SE$ (mg)	*n*
Saline			5.34±0.99	25
MK-801	1		2.46±4.04	17
t-PA	1	60	9.09±1.23*	11
MK-801 + t-PA	1 + 1	60	12.32±0.95**	12
MK-801 + t-PA	1 + 1	90	8.44±1.88	12

* Significantly different from control
** Significantly different from t-PA alone

Table 2. Interaction of anti-ICAM and t-PA

Group	Dose (mg/kg)	Time (min)	n	$ES_{50} \pm SE$ (mg)
Control			24	2.61±0.18
Anti-ICAM	2	15	17	3.03±0.37
t-PA	3	120	27	3.90±0.87
Anti-ICAM + t-PA	2 + 3	15 + 120	19	4.61±0.68*

* Significantly different from control

This model was also used to study combination therapy with an antiICAM monoclonal antibody plus rtPA. While the rtPA/MK-801 study was designed to increase the amount of clot the animal could tolerate, the rtPA/antiICAM study attempted to increase the window of time until start of treatment. Data showed that the combination could extend the time window to 2 hours, whereas neither drug alone was effective when treatment was initiated at 2 hours. This is evidence for a positive interaction of the combination (Table 2) [3].

These studies illustrate what can be gained from well designed preclinical trials of combinations. This approach is an effective and time efficient way of determining whether two drugs are likely to be useful, even if one or both lack efficacy as monotherapy, and it can serve as a reasonable basis for developing human clinical protocols.

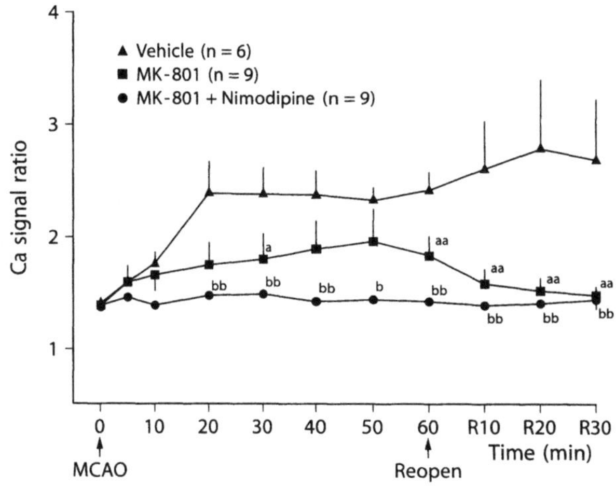

Fig. 2. Effect of reperfusion on calcium

Clinical Trials in Multimodality Therapy

J. Grotta

The complexity of the ischemic cascade suggests that a neuroprotective strategy affecting only one step is likely to produce only a modest clinical benefit. This should be reflected in future clinical trial design. For example, the restoration of perfusion after a prolonged time interval does not normalize calcium homeostasis unless a neuroprotective agent is administered during the ischemic interval [4]. Studies in a middle cerebral artery occlusion model showed that reperfusion did not restore calcium homeostasis and that intracellular calcium remained too high. Adding MKor MKand nimodipine blocked the calcium increase completely and maximized the benefits of reperfusion (Fig. 2).

A number of preclinical studies have shown that combinations of neuroprotection and reperfusion are effective. In recent work we were able to demonstrate that a combination of lubeluzole and diaspirin crosslinked hemoglobin (DCLHb) was effective in experimental ischemia [5]. DCLHb is a stable compound that does not dissociate and that has an oxygen affinity similar to blood. It can be given like saline without typing and without risk of infection. It appears to be a nearly ideal hemodiluting substance.

In our animal model of stroke blood was exchanged for 10% DCLHb to achieve a hematocrit reduction to about 30%. The infarct volume in treated animals was compared to that in animals who received albumin. In middle cerebral artery occlusion models there is a threshold beyond which time injury starts to appear. In this model the threshold is about an hour and a half of middle cerebral artery occlusion. Treating animals with DCLHb beginning 15 minutes after ischemia doubled the time before damage occurred. Albumin had no effect (Fig. 3). Adding lubeluzole to DCLHb actually decreased the size of the infarct produced by any given duration of ischemia that was tested (Fig. 4).

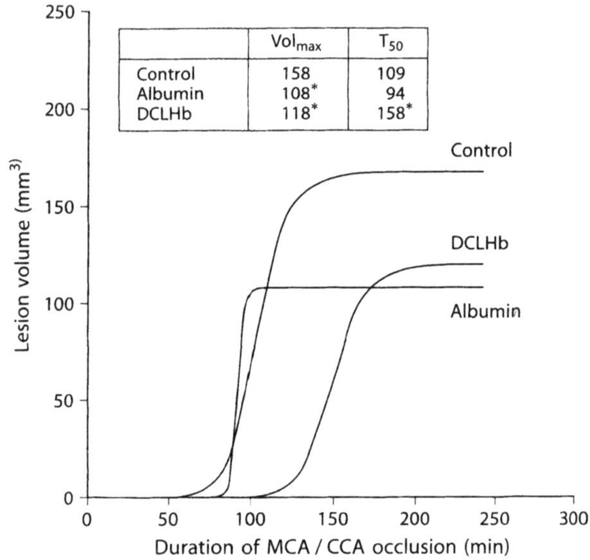

Fig. 3. Effect of DCLHb on time to infarct

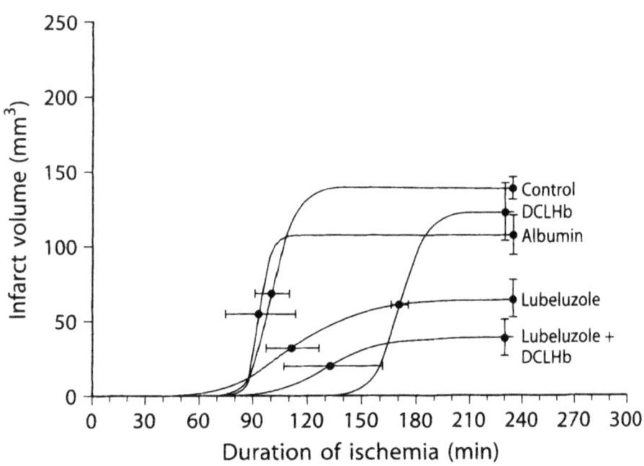

Fig. 4. Effect of lubeluzole and DCLHb on infarct volume

Thus, combining the two agents both prolongs the time before ischemia causes damage and reduces the magnitude of the damage that occurs. Together, these drugs have a substantial additive effect and would seem to warrant a clinical trial.

No human trials combining two or more therapeutic strategies for acute stroke are underway. There are a number of reasons for this situation. Laboratory impediments include the need for reproducible models of injury and the reluctance of pharmaceutical companies to fund work on combinations rather than evaluations of their drug alone. Pharmaceutical company impediments include the need to share profits of effective combinations, regulatory concerns, statistical concerns related to sample size, increased trial costs for testing combinations, and the need for collaboration between otherwise competing companies. These problems must be addressed before clinical trials of combination therapy can be expected to become a reality.

The impact of rtPA must also be considered. Since it has been approved in the U.S. for use within the first 3 hours after stroke onset, the logical next step would be to add it to other drugs being tested. That raises the question of interactions between rtPA and other drugs which might interfere with its thrombolytic activity or cause adverse effects. This needs to be tested in two-agent safety and efficacy studies in humans.

Conclusion

Combination therapy with neuroprotective and thrombolytic agents is rapidly emerging as the most promising avenue of care for acute stroke. A number of trials of singleagent neuroprotective therapy are underway. If trials seeking a prolonged time window are negative, these agents should still be considered for use in combination therapy trials and for trials within a shorter time window. Significant barriers to clinical trials of combination therapy remain, but the theoretical support for this approach from preclinical (animal) studies is unequivocal.

References

1. Zivin JA, deGirolami U, Kochhar A, et al (1987) A model for quantitative evaluation of embolic stroke therapy. Brain Res 435:305–309
2. Zivin JA, Mazzarella V (1991) Tissue plasminogen activator plus glutamate antagonist improves outcome after embolic stroke. Arch Neurol 48:1235–1238
3. Bowes MP, Rothlein R, Fagan SC, et al (1995) Monoclonal antibodies preventing leukocyte activation reduce experimental neurologic injury and enhance efficacy of thrombolytic therapy. Neurology 45:815–819
4. Uematsu D, Araki N, Greenberg JH, et al (1991) Combined therapy with MK-801 and nimodipine for protection of ischemic brain damage [see comments]. Neurology 41(1):88–94
5. Aronowski J, Strong R, Grotta JC: Combined neuroprotection and reperfusion therapy for stroke: the effect of lubeluzole and diaspirin crosslinked hemoglobin in experimental focal ischemia. Stroke 27:1571–1576

Medical Management of Elevated ICP

C. K. Spiss, U. M. Illievich, T. Shimizu, and G. Clifton

Introduction

The use of hypothermia, potentially in combination with recombinant tissue plasminogen activatase (rt-PA), is being explored for neuroprotective and thrombolytic application in the acute treatment of stroke. The beneficial effect of hypothermia appears to be due to effects on neurotransmitter release or reuptake or alterations in free radical scavenging activity. Clinical application of hypothermia must take into consideration potential adverse effects, including alterations in pharmacokinetics and pharmacodynamics of commonly used drugs. Results from ongoing clinical trials of hypothermia, including a multi-center study in acute traumatic brain injury, are expected to further define the therapeutic potential of this modality.

Hypothermia

Deliberate hypothermia has been used for decades as a therapeutic adjunct for various medical procedures, and deep global hypothermia is a principal component of circulatory arrest procedures. Specific effects of hypothermia on the various organ systems led to the development of a clinical temperature scale which defines mild hypothermia as body temperatures down to 34 °C, moderate as 34 to 28 °C, deep as 28 to 17 °C, and profound as 17 to 4°C [1]. Brain temperature decreases rapidly during cerebral ischemia unless temperature is actively maintained [2]. Histologic damage decreases substantially when the temperature drops from 36 to 33°C. Studies in severe head injury have shown that in patients with Glasgow Coma Scale less than 8, hypothermia reduces intracranial pressure (ICP), cerebral blood flow (CBF), and the cerebral metabolic rate (CMR), producing a trend toward improved morbidity and mortality [3–6].

Body temperature varies, both between different parts of the body and between the surface and the core. For practical purposes core temperature is used as a proxy for overall brain temperature However, if body core temperature is used to estimate cerebral temperature under nonischemic conditions, temperature gradients within the brain must also be considered. Temperature monitoring in the jugular bulb is invasive but is also a more precise measurement of brain temperature. Tympanic temperature, which is usually slightly lower than the temperature of the epidural space, can be used for noninvasive estimation of brain temperature so long as the surface of the head is not exposed to an extreme environment.

Body temperature is precisely regulated by thermoregulatory responses. Vasoconstriction as a thermoregulatory response to cold stress can be expected in sedated individuals with temperatures near 34 °C. This response is one that limits cutaneous heat loss. This diminishes the ability to achieve temperatures lower than that by surface cooling. We found that about 50% of patients vasoconstrict at 34.4 °C. The patients in whom vasoconstriction occurred required nearly an hour longer to reach a core temperature cooled to 32 °C.

Attenuating the thermoregulatory response is thus important for reaching the target temperature quickly. Circulating water and forced air cooling are the options available for most patients. Circulating water cooling is relatively inefficient because of little surface skin contact. Forced air cooling is more effective.

The initial hemodynamic pattern in patients with accidental deep hypothermia showed a marked hypovolemia with a simultaneous decrease of both cardiac output and ventricular filling pressure, and a decreased total blood volume [7]. The conduction system in the myocardium is more sensitive to cold, so the cardiac cycle is lengthened and bradycardia occurs. We have investigated the effect of graded hypothermia on hemodynamics, oxygen kinetics, and myocardial wall motion and found luxury perfusion (Fig. 1).

Rewarming can cause problems because it places demands on the cardiovascular system. Shivering is not only uncomfortable but also dangerous because it increases cardiac output and increases total body oxygen consumption. The associated higher myocardial oxygen demand may induce myocardial ischemia in some patients [8]. Therefore, rewarming speed must be very slow.

Side effects of hypothermia are also a concern. There are two reasons to suspect that hypothermia facilitates development of postoperative wound infection. The first is thermoregulatory vasoconstriction, which leads to low tissue partial oxygen pressure persisting long after restoration of normothermia, and reduced production of bactericidal superoxide radicals. The second is reduced immune function, including leukocyte mobility and phagocytosis, T-cell mediated antibody production, and release of immune mediators.

Hypothermia can also interfere with monitoring equipment. Neuromuscular blockade can produce misleading electromyograms. For this reason we monitor

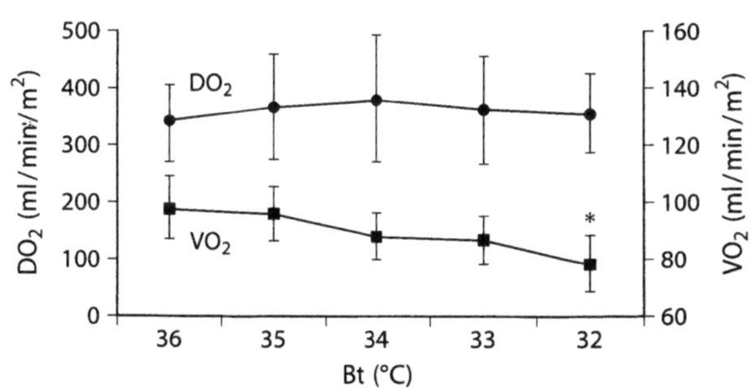

Fig. 1. Hemodynamic changes in deep hypothermia

neuromuscular block by following mechanical twitch tension. Finger pulse oximetry may fail, and alternative measuring sites such as the nose should be considered.

Because hypothermia affects both the activation and the basal metabolism of neuronal cells, it may also interfere with neurophysiological monitoring. As temperature drops from 36 °C to 31 °C, there is a significant increase in the central conduction time of the SSEP from 6.8 msec to almost 9 msec (Fig. 2). Similar delays occur in the auditory evoked potentials.

Monitoring cerebral electrical function can be performed. The results are less helpful due to variability. We find that electroencephalograms may shift toward slower frequencies, and the latencies and amplitude of somatosensory evoked potentials (SSEP) may vary.

Hypothermia also alters the pharmacokinetics and pharmacodynamics of inhalation anesthetics. MAC decreases by 5% per degree C. Solubility of anesthesia increases. Partial pressure is unchanged, so there is no net increase of anesthetic effect [9]. Decreased metabolism prolongs the action of muscle relaxants. For example, for vecuronium a two-degree temperature reduction doubles the duration of pharmacologic effect. Decreased metabolism also increases propofol plasma concentrations such that a three-degree temperature reduction causes a 30% increase in concentration.

Hypothermia affects the acid-base balance because gas becomes less soluble at lower temperatures. Blood pH increases 0.015 pH units for every degree of temperature decrease. There are two approaches to maintaining the patient's acid-base status during hypothermia: pH stat or alpha stat. PH stat management varies $PaCO_2$ to maintain the correct pH. The use of pH stat management in hypothermia will result in a relative brain tissue acidosis and abolition of cerebral blood flow autoregulation. Lower metabolic rates are associated with decreased CO_2 production, which may lead to respiratory alkalosis when ventilation in the paralyzed patient is not changed accordingly. Alpha stat management keeps the uncorrected pH as measured at 37 °C constant and preserves autoregulation [10]. This effect is based on the dissociation state of the alpha imidazole ring on histidine.

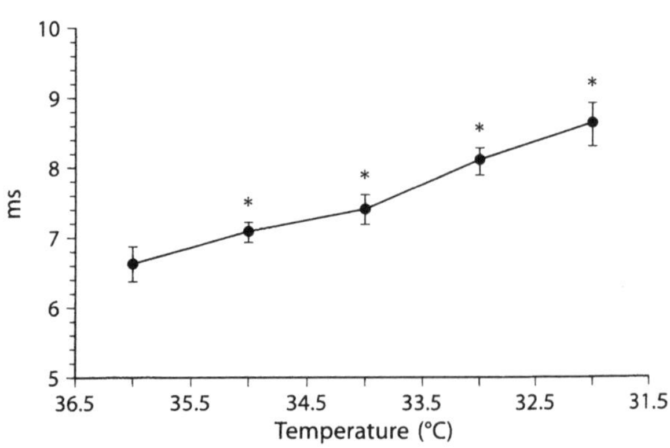

Fig. 2. SSEP central conduction time and hypothermia

Alpha stat is named after the dissociation state of the alpha imidazole ring of histidine. This group functions as an important buffer of hemoglobin and other body proteins. For optimal enzyme function it is important to maintain a constant imidazole ionization. The ratio (alpha) of dissociated to undissociated imidazole groups stays constant (alpha stat) during temperature reduction.

Hypothermia is associated with coagulation disorders. These include reversible platelet sequestration, reversible platelet dysfunction due to reduced thromboxane A2 activity, reduced enzyme activity leading to prolonged clotting and bleeding times, and perhaps increased fibrinolysis. The influence of hypothermia on coagulation has been studied in cardiopulmonary bypass patients, in plasma obtained at normothermia but analyzed at hypothermia, and in plasma from hypothermic patients analyzed at hypothermia [11–13]. These studies are difficult to compare due to different investigative protocols.

Over the last decades numerous in vitro and animal studies indicate a potential adverse effect of hypothermia on the hemostasis system [14–16]. However, besides study protocols with induced coagulopathies, e.g. cardiopulmonary bypass or trauma, there are differences in species, grade and extent (local or global) of hypothermia and assay temperature. One problem of in vitro studies is that they only reflect a part of the changes that decreased body temperature has on the coagulation and fibrinolytic system. These tests do not consider other in vivo changes in hypothermic subjects like the increase in blood viscosity and alterations of the balance between the fluid phase and the vessel wall. Furthermore, the clearance of activated factors and the production of proteins relevant for the balance between coagulation and fibrinolysis by the liver is neglected. Therefore, these results allow only limited conclusions regarding the hemostasis system in humans with a body temperature between 36 and 32 °C. Although the possibility of a hypothermia-induced coagulopathy has not yet been excluded in patients with severe head injuries, the short-term use of hypothermia does not appear to increase the risk for intracranial hemorrhagic complications in these patients [17].

We studied the effects of hypothermia in on coagulation state. Baseline values were obtained 24 hours prior to the study. Blood was drawn at 36 °C, 34 °C, and 32 °C.

We found that moderate hypothermia (32 °C) does not change basal coagulation activity, does not activate fibrinolysis, and does not cause endothelial stress in anesthetized humans [14].

We used transcranial Doppler (TCD) ultrasound to investigate cerebral blood flow velocity during hypothermia. When patients were cooled to 32 °C there was a reduction in CBF velocity from about 50 cm/sec to about 30 cm/sec (Fig. 3). However, the CO_2 handling ability was unaffected.

The classic mechanism, a temperature dependent decrease of oxygen and glucose metabolism as the sole mediator by which hypothermia provides protection from ischemia has lately been challenged. Several animal studies have now demonstrated, that mild degrees of hypothermia (2 °–4 °C temperature reduction) are associated with substantial effects on histologic damage. The neuroprotective ef-

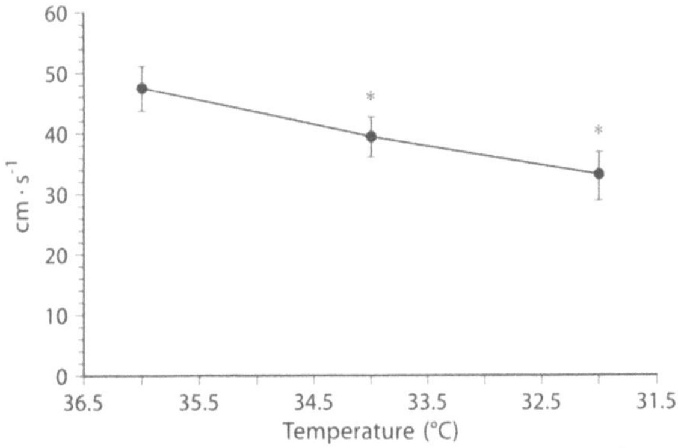

Fig. 3. Effect of hypothermia on cerebral blood flow velocity

fect of mild and moderate hypothermia is based on interactions with many steps of the ischemic cascade. We suspect that mild hypothermia may protect the brain by altering the release or reuptake of neurotransmitters such as glutamate or aspartate or by changing free radical production or scavenging. Hypothermia has been shown to decrease the glutamate response to ischemia more than isoflurane, pentobarbital, or propofol (Fig. 4) [15]. Details of protection from free radical mediated injury remain to be evaluated.

One potential free radical mechanism of a hypothermic protective effect is the influence of hypothermia on ion flux. In ischemia in the absence of hypothermia, sodium and chloride influxes are followed by water influx and cell swelling. Potassium efflux is followed by membrane depolarization. Calcium ion accumulation activates proteases and phospholipases A1, A2, and C. The result is destruction of cell membranes, receptor dysfunction, hydrolysis of membrane phospholipids, membrane disruption, and release of free fatty acids. We think hypother-

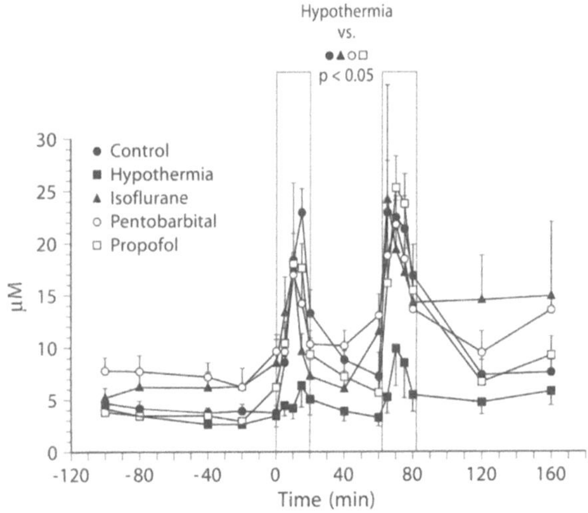

Fig. 4. Effect of hypothermia on glutamate

mia protects the brain by alterations in ion homeostasis (including calcium and potassium fluxes), increased membrane stability (including the blood-brain barrier), and decreased enzyme function (including phospholipase and xanthine oxidase). This decreased enzyme function could well be associated with decreased production of toxic metabolites such as free radicals.

However, there are still unanswered questions. We are awaiting the results of trials to demonstrate efficacy. We are not sure about the cost-benefit ratio for hypothermia therapies. Questions remain about the optimal temperature, measurement sites, and best methods of cooling and rewarming.

Combined Hypothermia and Thrombolysis

Experimental studies have thus demonstrated the importance of brain temperature in the pathophysiology of cerebral ischemia. We have conducted two studies that examined issues related to body temperature in acute stroke patients. The first, done in collaboration with Wataru Kakuda, examined effects without active hypothermic intervention. The first study included retrospective analysis of data on 60 patients (30 male, 30 female, 17 to 94 y.o. averaged 68 ± 31 years) with cardiogenic embolism. They had been admitted at 1 to 24 hours after stroke, average 10 ± 14 hours. CT scan was performed serially to evaluate the severity of cerebral edema, occurrence of hemorrhagic transformation, and infarct size. Body temperature was monitored at the axilla using a thermometer. The temperature measurements were performed 6 times a day during the first 7 days after admission. The mean body temperature during the first 3 days was used to classify patients into 3 groups. The frequency of severe edema and hemorrhagic transformation and of large infarcts was compared among these three groups. The second study was an intervention to clarify the effects of mild hypotension on embolic stroke. The second study included 5 patients with cardiogenic embolism. rt-PA had been given to 4 patients but occluded vessels could not be completely reopened. The fifth patient was admitted at 24 hours after onset and did not receive rt-PA. Patients were cooled to 33 °C and maintained for 3 to 7 days using hypothermia blankets and alcohol spray. Plain and enhanced CT scans were performed serially. The size of cerebral infarct, severity of brain edema, occurrence of hemorrhagic transformation, and existence of contrast enhancement were evaluated. Clinical outcome was also evaluated.

The effects of body temperature in the acute phase of ischemic injury was studied in 60 cases of cardiogenic embolism. Patients were evaluated for body temperature control within the first 24 hours of stroke onset. Patients were divided into three groups based on average body temperature during the first 3 days after stroke. These were >37.0 °C ($n=11$), 36.5–37.0 °C ($n=33$), and <36.5 °C ($n=16$).

The size of infarction, grade of cerebral edema, and presence or absence of hemorrhagic transformation were evaluated from delayed computed tomography (CT). CT scan was executed twice at least. The CT on admission and the follow-up CT performed at 3 to 14 days after stroke were analyzed.

Almost 50% (6/11) patients with average temperature >37.0 °C had severe cerebral edema. None of the patients with temperature <36.5 °C had severe edema. Likewise, 9 of 11 patients in the first group had hemorrhagic transformation, but only 2 of 14 patients in the group with the lowest temperatures experienced hemorrhagic transformation. All of the patients in the highest temperature group had large infarctions involving areas larger than the middle cerebral artery territory. None of the patients in the lowest-temperature group had such large infarctions.

Thus, even a small difference in body temperature in the acute phase seems to affect the grade of edema, hemorrhagic transformation, and focal size of infarction. However, this observational study does not indicate whether high body temperature is the cause or the result of severe injury.

To address this question, the effects of applying mild hypothermia therapy during the acute phase of cerebral ischemia were studied in 5 cases of cardiogenic embolism. Cases 1–4 were admitted within 4 hours of the stroke. All had occlusion of the internal carotid artery or middle cerebral artery and all were treated with rt-PA immediately after admission. Cases 1 and 4 had partial reopenings of the artery 3 hours and 8 hours after stroke, respectively. Cases 2 and 3 had no reopening. Case 5 was referred 24 hours after stroke and did not receive rt-PA.

Hypothermia was initiated within 6 hours after stroke in cases 1–4 and 24 hours after stroke in case 5. Hypothermia was continued for 3 days in cases 1,2, and 4, for 5 days in case 3, and for 7 days in case 5. The effects of treatment were evaluated on the basis of CT findings and clinical outcome.

Figure 4 demonstrates the results of case 2, a 68-year-old male. At 7 hours after stroke the patient continued to have occlusion of the right middle cerebral artery (Fig. 5A). Serial CT scans, however, showed almost no appreciable ischemic lesion, in spite of the prominent occlusion of the middle cerebral artery (Fig. 5B). This patient was discharged without neurological deficit.

Case 5 showed the most dramatic CT findings and clinical course (Fig. 6A–C). This 16-year old girl had open-heart surgery and did not wake up from a comatose state for almost one day. CT scan performed 24 hours after surgery and before hypothermia demonstrated cerebral edema and right cerebral hemisphere shift of midline structure toward the contralateral side. The cardiac surgeon suspected brain death was likely to occur but applied hypothermia therapy. After the start of hypothermia CT showed gradual amelioration of cerebral edema. The shift of midline structures disappeared almost completely. Contrast enhancement CT performed 4 days after stroke, at which time cerebral edema still remained severe, showed low parenchymal enhancement in the ischemic area. Presumably, normal blood-brain barrier function was restored by the hypothermia. This patient showed an excellent symptomatic recovery. She began to walk with a cane 4 months after stroke and returned to high school with excellent grades.

CT findings of hemorrhagic changes are summarized in Fig. 7. Cases 1, 2, 3, and 5 had no hemorrhagic changes. Case 4 had minor hemorrhagic conversion immediately after the start of hypothermia and additional changes thereafter.

Clinical outcomes were excellent (Table 1). Neurological deficits were absent or moderate in cases 1–4. All could walk without aid. Case 5 had definite hemipare-

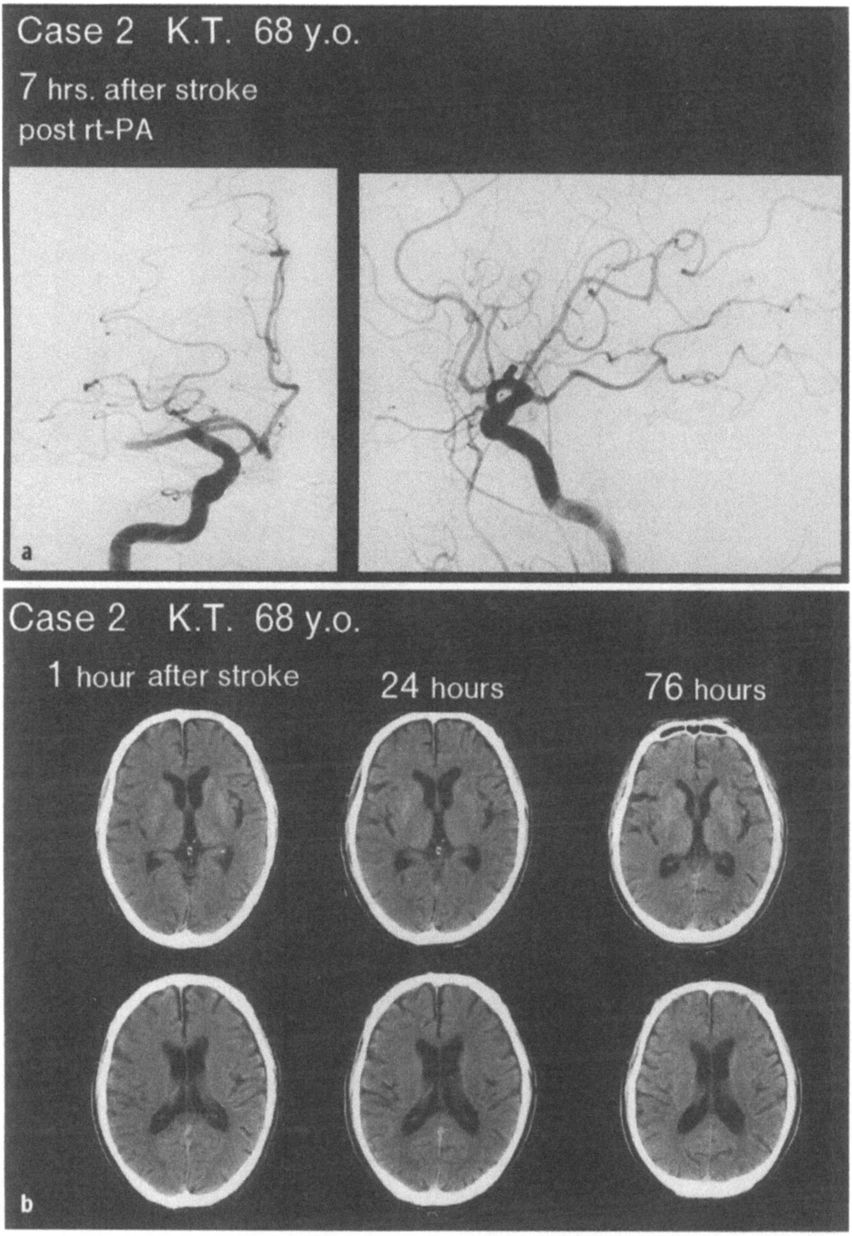

Fig. 5. **a** Angiography of occlusion in case 2. **b** Serial CT showing lack of ischemic damage in case 2

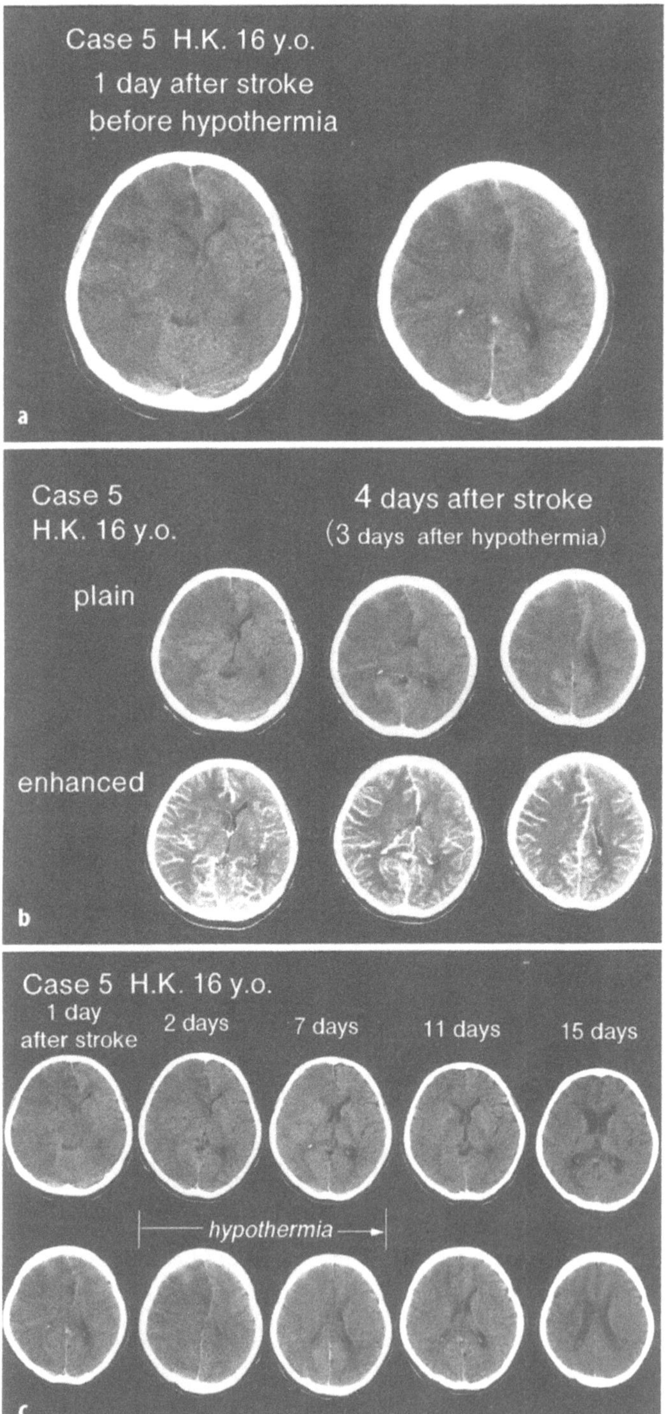

Fig. 6. a Case 5 one day after stroke, before hypothermia. **b** Serial CT of case 5. **c** Enhancement CT of case 5 4 days after stroke

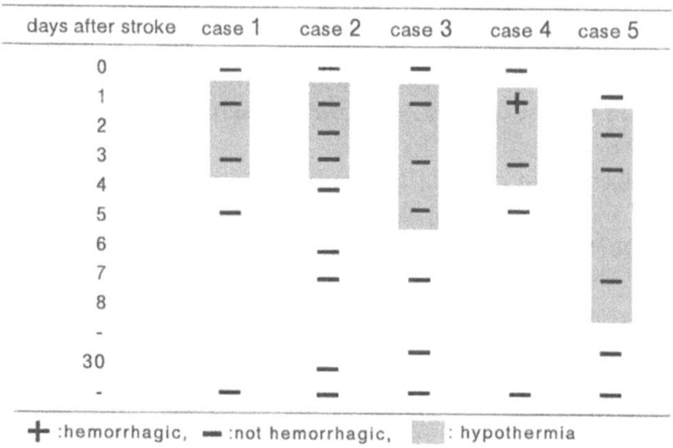

Fig. 7. Hemorrhagic changes on CT

Table 1. Clinical outcome

	Infarct size	Neurological deficit	Gait
1	Medium	Mild aphasia, hand clumsiness	Normal
2	Trivial	None	Normal
3	Large	Mild aphasia, moderate hemiparesis	Without aid
4	Small	Mild hemiparesis	Without aid
5	Large	Hemiparesis	With aid

sis, but her recovery from the comatose state was unexpected and greatly appreciated by both the patient and her family.

This small series suggests the potential usefulness of mild hypothermic therapy in acute stroke. The effectiveness of such therapy is most likely represented by three characteristic CT findings in this series: absence of appreciable edema or mass effect, rare occurrence of hemorrhagic transformation, and absence of enhancement on contrast CT. These findings apparently indicate that the blood-brain-barrier function remains intact. Since this is largely determined by the endothelium, the CT findings suggest that mild hypothermia protects the endothelium from ischemic injury.

NABIS-H: The North American Hypothermia in Acute Traumatic Brain Injury Study

The North American Hypothermia in Acute Traumatic Brain Injury Study is a multicenter study of systemic hypothermia in severe brain injury begun in 1994 and funded by the U. S. National Institutes of Health. The study includes patients in Houston, Sacramento, Pittsburgh, Indianapolis, Detroit, Boston, Dallas, Camden, and St. Louis. Mean age of patients is 32.1 years, and about 75% of patients are male.

Inclusion criteria are Glasgow Coma Scale motor score of 1–5, non-penetrating head injury, GCS of 3–8 after resuscitation (1.5 hours after admission), and ages 16–65 years.

Exclusion criteria are inability to initiate cooling within 6 hours after injury, GCS 7–8 with a normal CT scan or a CT scan showing only minimal (<2 mm) subarachnoid hemorrhage or a skull fracture, systolic blood pressure <90 mmHg for >30 minutes post-resuscitation, or O_2 saturation <94% for >30 minutes post resuscitation.

The objective is to cool the patient to 33 °C within 8 hours of injury. Cooling lasts for 48 hours. Patients are then warmed very slowly, about half a degree every two hours. patients are randomized either in the emergency room or in the operating room.

The protocol calls for 500 patients and has the power to detect a 10% difference in Glasgow Outcome Scale (GCS) at 6 months after injury.

One problem observed in the pilot study was that many patients are hypothermic at presentation. We elected not to rewarm any patients but to assess GCS at the presenting temperature. After randomization, if the patient is assigned to hyperthermia, there is further cooling to 33 °C. Patients randomized to the normothermic arm warm themselves by application of non-heated, insulated blankets. Cooling is to maintain Foley temperature at 32–33.5 °C. Gastric ice water lavage by nasogastric tube is done until temperature is less than 33.5 °C. Rotorest bed with hypothermia blanket attachment is wrapped around the patient and set in automatic mode at 32.7 °C.

Fluid management includes total fluid replacement plus estimated insensible losses. No dextrose is given IV except for total parenteral nutrition (TPN).

For ICP management, if ventriculostomy is present, 1 ml of cerebrospinal fluid (CSF) is drained per minute up to 6 ml per hour. Morphine and vencuronium are given for paralysis, sedation, and analgesia. Mannitol is given until ICP remains <20 or serum osmolality is 315 milliosmols. If osmolality is over 315, mannitol is held and status is checked every 2 hours. Hyperventilation is used with a goal of maintaining $PaCO_2$ over 25. When a patient does not respond to these measures barbiturate therapy is given.

If patients meet the ICP criterion but serum osmolality is over 315, they are given barbiturates. Pentobarbital is given at 10 mg/kg loading dose, the rate being guided by cardiovascular response. During the first 15 minutes of each subsequent hour pentobarbital is given at 5 mg/kg and adjusted to maintain a serum level of 30–40 mcg/dl. Vasopressors and volume expansion are used to maintain a cerebral perfusion pressure of >70 mmHg during barbiturate usage.

Nutritional management in the normothermia arm is to begin enteral or parenteral feeding within 48 hours of admission, with jejunal feedings recommended. Patients in the hypothermia arm begin enteral or parenteral feeding when the patient's temperature reaches 37 °C (72 hours after admission).

Thus far 180 patients have been randomized and follow-up is 97%. Measures to maximize follow-up include patient reimbursement, use of a brief 1.5-hr psychologic test battery, funding to fly outcome personnel to the patient for assessment, and frequent patient contact by the study nurse. The study is expected to be completed in 1999.

Conclusion

As emergency treatment of acute stroke moves toward incorporating neuroprotective and thrombolytic therapies, hypothermia is attracting greater clinical interest. Issues of optimal clinical application and avoiding adverse effects remain unresolved, but there is preliminary evidence that moderate hypothermia will have a place in the emergency management of acute stroke.

References

1. Hitchcock CR, Strobel CJA, Haglin JJ, et al (1962) Use of prolonged moderate hypothermia in postoperative care. Arch Surg 85:549–556
2. Busto R, Dietrich WD, Globus MY, et al (1987) Small differences in intraischemic brain temperature critically determine the extent of ischemic neuronal injury. J Cereb Blood Flow Metab 7:729–738
3. Marion DW, Obrist WD, Carlier PM, et al (1993) The use of moderate therapeutic hypothermia for patients with severe head injuries: a preliminary report. J Neurosurg 79:354–362
4. Clifton GL, Allen S, Barrodale P, et al (1993) A phase II study of moderate hypothermia in severe brain injury. J Neurotrauma 10:263–271
5. Shiozake T, Sugimoto H, Taneda M, et al (1993) Effect of mild hypothermia on uncontrollable intracranial hypertension after severe head injury. J Neurosurgery 79:363–368
6. Marion DW, Penrod LE, Kelsey SF, et al (1997) Treatment of traumatic brain injury with moderate hypothermia. N Engl J Med 336:540–546
7. Harari A, Regnier B, Rapin M et al (1975) Haemodynamic study of prolonged deep accidental hypothermia. Eur J Intensive Care Med 1:65–70
8. Frank SM, Beattie C, Christopherson R, et al (1993) Unintentional hypothermia is associated with postoperative myocardial ischemia. The Perioperative Ischemia Randomized Anesthesia Trial Study Group. Anesthesiology 78:468–476
9. Eger EII, Johnson BH (1987) MAC of I-653 in rats, including a test of the effect of body temperature and anesthetic duration. Anesth Analg 66:974–976
10. Verhaegen MJ, Todd MM, Hindman BJ, et al (1993) Cerebral autoregulation during moderate hypothermia in rats. Stroke 24:407–414
11. Patt A, McCroskey BL, Moore EE (1988) Hypothermia-induced coagulopathies in trauma. Surg Clin North Am 68:775–785
12. Rohrer MJ, Natale AM (1992) Effect of hypothermia on the coagulation cascade. Crit Care Med 20:1402–1405
13. Reed RL, Johnson TD, Hudson JD, et al (1992) The disparity between hypothermic coagulopathy and clotting studies. J Trauma 33:465–470
14. Sitzwohl C, Kozek S, Kapiotis S, et al (1996) Effect of graded hypothermia (36 °C–32 °C) on basal activity of the coagulation and fibrinolytic system. Anesthesiology 85:A168
15. Illievich UM, Zornow MH, Choi KT, et al (1994) Effects of hypothermia or anesthetics on hippocampal glutamate and glycine concentrations after repeated transient global cerebral ischemia. Anesthesiology 80:177–186
16. Wilson JT, Miller WR (1958) Blood studies in the hypothermic dog. Surgery 43:979–989
17. Resnick DK, Marion DW, Darby JM (1994) The effect of hypothermia on the incidence of delayed traumatic intracerebral hemorrhage. Neurosurgery 34:252–255

Surgical Management of Elevated ICP and Monitoring

T. Steiner and A. Aschoff

Introduction

The clinical characteristics of space occupying hemispheric infarction might be described as severe hemispheric stroke syndrome involving the territory of the middle and/or anterior cerebral artery with hemiplegia and forced eye and head deviation on admission. This is followed by progressive deterioration of consciousness within 2–3 days [1]. The progression of symptoms is produced by brain edema within the first days, with a maximum occurring on day 3 to 5 [2]. Clinically this mass effect presents as ipsilateral pupillary dilatation [3] (19 out of 35) and death within 2 to 5 days due to increased intracranial pressure with transtentorial herniation (25 out of 35) [4]. Because of the rapid development of cerebral edema with subsequent herniation we have suggested to use the term "malignant" MCA (middle cerebral artery) infarction [1].

The mortality of malignant MCA infarction is between 40% [5,6]. Physical and pharmacological conservative treatments often fail to control elevated intracranial pressure (ICP). Decompressive hemicraniectomy has been reported to be an effective lifesaving procedure and to improve the unfavorable outcome in this group of patients [7–11]. The practice of decompressive craniectomy is based on the assumption that the procedure can improve perfusion of leptomeningeal collaterals, improve retrograde perfusion of the MCA, optimize cerebral perfusion of the ischemic penumbra, and by this reduce infarction size and consequent reduce neurological deficit [12, 13].

We started an ongoing prospective trial in 1990 on patients with massive cerebral infarction. This trial should answer the following questions: Do people with space occupying hemispheric infarction benefit from decompressive surgery? What other factors might influence the outcome? Does the initial clinical status give a hint towards the course of the disease? Does timing of intervention play a role concerning the outcome?

We included patients with right hemispheric stroke syndrome who are younger than 70 years, and whose preoperative CCT shows a space occupying hemispheric infarction with midline shift of at least 5 mm at the septum pellucidum level or a shift of the pineal gland, compressed basal cisterns, or uncal herniation. In every case we required signed informed consent. We excluded patients older than 70 years, with complete global aphasia and/or with secondary parenchymal hemorrhage.

A control group included patients who had infarction of the dominant hemisphere, and had additional severe medical complications that increased the perioperative risk, and or were unable to give informed consent.

Standard Treatment Protocol

Our standardized treatment includes basic medical therapy and antiedema treatment (Table 1). We give sedation and artificial ventilation in case of progressing clinical deterioration. We hyperventilate all patients with crisis elevation of ICP [14, 15].

Our standard monitoring protocol consists of serial CCT, routine and diagnostic vascular studies, and evoked potentials at least in all ventilated patients [16]. Continuous ICP monitoring is the ideal goal but not always possible [5,6].

To date we have completed statistics in 57 treated patients. Thirty patients with malignant MCA infarction were not operated during the same study period.

Table 1. Peri-operative, conservative therapy in patients with space occupying massive cerebral infarction

General basic therapy	
Blood pressure control	RR_{sys}120 to 160 mmHg, RR_{dias} 60 to 90mmHg*
Blood glucose	$\leq$120 mg/dl
Body temperature	$\leq$37 °C
Avoid hypoxia	keep paO_2 >90 mmHg
Avoid hyperkapnia	keep 35 mmHg $\leq paCO_2 \leq$ 45 mmHg
Basic antiedematous therapy	
Elevated head positioning	Following the clinical picture or ICP monitoring
Glycerol	50% p.o.: 4 × 50 to 100 ml/day 10% i.v.: 4 × 125 to 250 ml/day (keep serum osmolarity <320 mmol/l)
Deterioration of consciousness with danger of aspiration and hypoventilation	Analgosedation, intubation, relaxation e.g., fentanyl, midazolam, succinyl
Treatment of crisis elevation of ICP	
Mannitol 20%	i.v.: up to 3 to 4 × 100 ml/d (keep serum osmolarity <320 mmol/l, *cave:* "rebound")
Hyper-HAES 7%	i.v.: 250 ml over 15 min keep serum osmolarity <320 mmol/l, Serum sodium < 155 mmol/l)
TRIS buffer	i.v.-Bolus: 1 mmol/kg BW, if succesful continued with 0.25 mmol/kg BW/h (central venous catheter)
Hyperventilation	30 mmHg $\leq pCO_2 \leq$ 35 mmHg
Short-acting barbiturates	E.g., thiopental, methohexital *cave*: cardiodepressive effects

* Depending on past medical history of hypertension

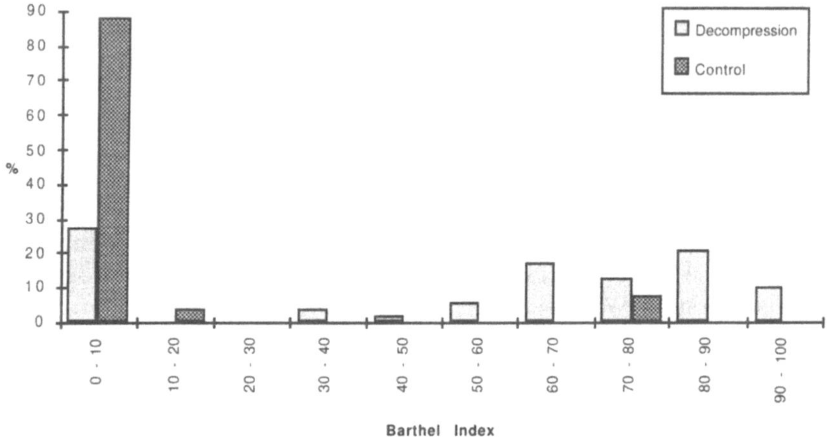

Fig. 1. Comparison of Barthel Scores

The biggest difference between the two groups was in mortality, which was 28% in the craniectomy group and 72% in the control group. Barthel-Index scores (BI) were not very well reflected by means. Figure 1 shows the distribution of BI scores comparing decompression with control. Sixty-one percent of patients who had surgery had BI scores between 60 and 90 points. On the other hand, 87% of patients who were treated conservatively had BI scores of 0 to 10 points. BI scores greater than 60 are regarded as slightly to not dependent on external help with activities of daily living.

Since the BI score does not reflect the degree of neurologic deficit, we also included the modified Rankin Scale (mRS). Figure 2 shows that 60% of the operat-

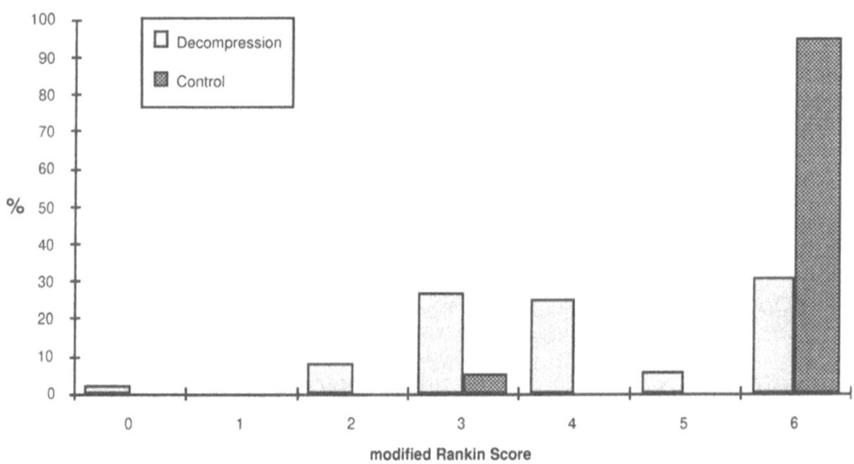

Fig. 2. Comparison of Rankin Scores

ed patients had mRS of 2 to 4, indicating mild to moderately severe disabled patients, whereas 84% of the control group had mRS of 6 (meaning that these patients died). These numbers indicate a further improvement of outcomes compared to those we have published in 1995 when Rieke et al demonstrated a decrease of mortality to below 35%, with the majority of operated patients having BI around 60 [5].

Monitoring of Patients and Prediction of Outcome

It is the nature of this disease that clinical assessment is limited at a certain point when analgosedation and ventilation become necessary. At this stage technical monitoring becomes inevitable.

Neuroradiologic imaging studies in the early phase of the disease can provide prognostic information: Analysis of 620 CCTs from the ECASS study revealed an increased relative risk for severe brain swelling if early infarction signs show that more than 33% of the MCA territory is involved. Relative risk was 6.64 and 5.4 in the placebo and rtPA groups, respectively.

Early infarct signs can be seen on the initial CCT in 68% of patients at two hours after onset of stroke and in 89% at the third hour [17]. Major infarct signs will become visible during the first 12 hours after onset of symptoms including severe brain swelling with midline shift. The positive predictive value for fatal outcome is 85%, if CCT hypodensity covers more than 50% of the MCA territory. The risk of fatal outcome is 70% if local brain swelling occurs in patients with angiographically proven MCA trunk occlusion [18].

Poor collateral blood supply and absence of recanalization within 8 to 24 hours after onset of symptoms induce further increase of ischemic edema and midline shift [18] (Fig. 3). Craniectomy lowered infarct size and improved outcome in an animal model, probably by improving collateral blood supply [13, 19]. Patients with malignant MCAinfarction suffer either from distal ICA (internal carotid artery) or proximal MCA/ACA (anterior cerebral artery) occlusion. In both situations collateral blood flow is diminished [20, 21]. Consequently, angiographically detected thrombus located at the distal ICA- or combined MCA-ACA in the may early predict malignant MCA infarction.

Unfortunately, these imaging and vascular studies are not suitable for continuous monitoring of rapidly developing brain edema. ICP monitoring does not have this disadvantage. It is also technically less demanding and less expensive. However, there are several problems with ICP guided therapy. First is the question of what pressure to treat? Though there has been no controlled study demonstrating the necessity of treatment at a certain ICP elevation, it is widespread habit to regard ICP values above 30 mmHg as indication for antiematose treatment. Clinical experience shows that some patients survive ICP's above 30 mmHg, and others die without reaching an ICP elevation of 30 mmHg. Other problems might rise from the probe's location. We found remarkable hydrostatic pressure influences on a-p pressure up to 11 mmHg (Fig. 4) and during side positioning of the head of ±4 mmHg. The potential addition of these effects might

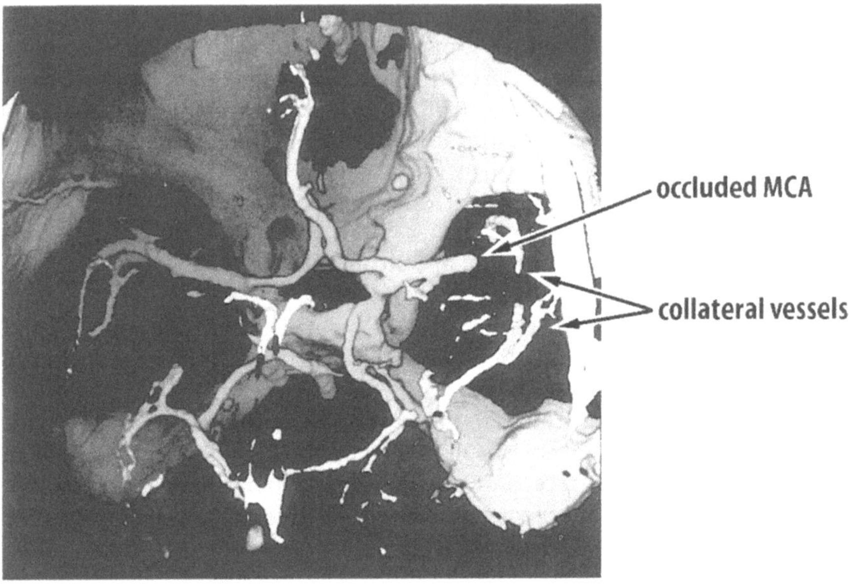

Fig. 3. Three dimensional reconstruction of CT-angiography showing MCA occlusion and collateral blood flow

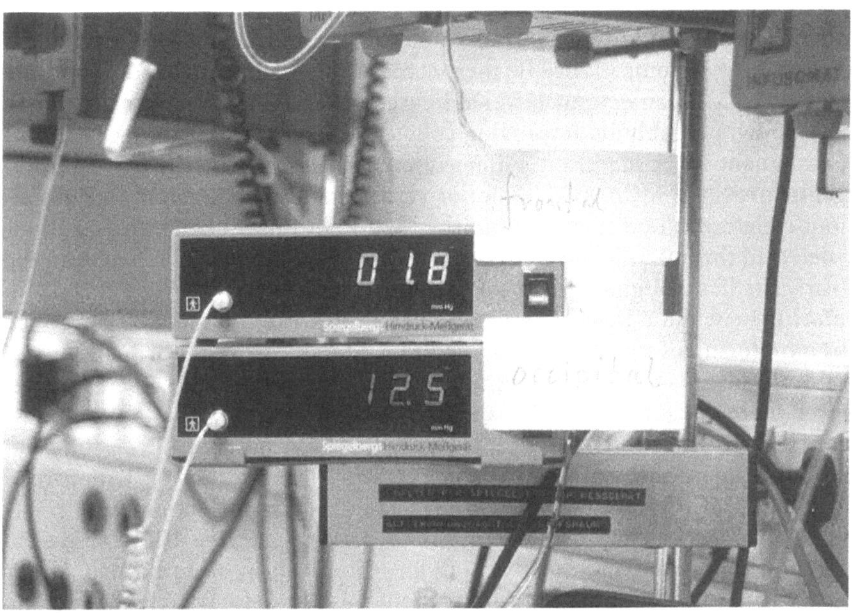

Fig. 4. Frontal and occipital epidural ICP measurement demonstrating the remarkable a–p pressure difference

erroneously lead to a situation regarded as "must be treated". Furthermore, ICP as it is measured today, is limited to regional use.

Whether single-sided ICP measurements are sufficient to monitor brain edema is still questionable. Given that there are significant variations an individual tolerance to CPP (cerebral perfusion pressures), there also remains the question of pressure (whether ICP or CPP) to treat at? We think from the pathophysiological point of view, the CPP is the more valuable parameter for guiding therapy of elevated ICP. Most authors recommend keeping CPP above 60 or even 70 mmHg [22–25]. Since CPP is defined by MAP (middle arterial pressure) and ICP, it is absolutely necessary to control the quality of the MAP and ICP measurement.

From this follows that it would be nice to have further online modalities, that help improve the clinical assessment of acute ICP changes. We have therefore started to monitor the cerebral $ptiO_2$ (partial tissue oxygen pressure) and CBF (cerebral blood flow). These two modalities are part of new protocols which have been proven by our ethical committee. We hypothesize that critical ICP elevations are correlated with measurable decreases in $ptiO_2$ and CBF.

$PtiO_2$ is measured with a microprobe within the white matter of the frontal lobe within the hemisphere contralateral to the infarcted side. ICP is measured on both hemispheres. $PtiO_2$ measurements have been performed in 10 patients with malignant MCA infarction. Decompressive surgery was performed in six patients. Of the 4 patients that died, one had received decompressive surgery. In 3 surviving patients we observed a decrease of $ptiO_2$ before surgery. After surgery, $ptiO_2$ returned to normal in all 3 patients. This was correlated with an increase of CPP and a decrease of ICP after surgery (Fig. 5) [26].

CBF is calculated by a double dye dilution technique with two combined fiber optic thermistor catheters in the right jugular bulb and the aorta. Fifty nine CBF measurements were performed in 8 patients. All 20 CBF values <30 ml/100 g/min were associated with corresponding clinical events (ICP

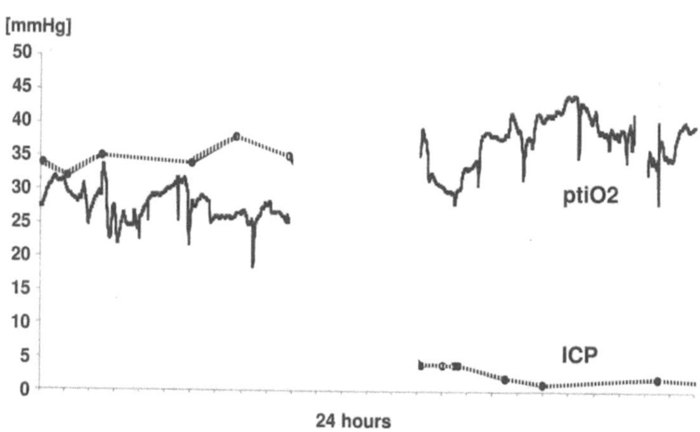

Fig. 5. ICP and $ptiO_2$ before and after hemicraniectomy

>20 mmHg, pupillary dilatation, brain herniation within 24 hours, hyperventilation). Patients who died showed low CBF values more often than patients who survived. CBF dropped during hyperventilation (except just preventing brain herniation), THAMBuffer and occasionally during elevated ICP. In terms of complications, we have had no infections or bleedings with these methods [27].

Craniectomy

Problems of decompressive craniectomy in space occupying infarction arise if the diameter is to small. This is because herniation at the edges of the skull may lead to compression of cortical veins, leading to an increase of ICP and possibly intracranial hemorrhage. Local intracerebral sheering forces, especially at the white grey matter border, may further lead to intracerebral bleedings. This typically occurs in close relation to the edges of the skull. On the other hand, the bigger the craniectomy area, the bigger the wound, with the increasing probability of wound bleedings and infections. Also, the bigger the problems with stability and brain positioning on the bed.

Craniectomies have a long tradition especially in neuro traumatology. Astonishing enough, there are no larger systematic or prospective trials on the correlation between volume effect and size of craniectomy. We therefor studied this relation using a spherical and cylindrical mathematical model which were defined as follows:

$$V_{\text{spherecut}} = \frac{\pi h \times h}{3} \ (3r - h)_{(\text{sphere cut})}$$

$$V_{\text{cylinder}} = \pi r h \times r_{(\text{cylinder})}$$

The assumption was made of a 50% correction of 15 mm from the ridge and a bone thickness of 6 mm. We found that there is a nearly logarithmic correlation between the diameter and the herniation effect. This is illustrated in Fig. 6. Though volumes differ slightly through the two models, it can be seen that diameters of 5 to 7 cm result in a gain of volume of only 3 to 13 ml. Effective herniations of about 100 ml are reached at diameters of 13 to 14 cm depending on the model.

A retrospective analyses of 48 of our hemicraniectomies revealed a mean diameter of 10.4 cm and a mean decompressive volume 66.5 ml. We could not demonstrate a difference between survivors and nonsurvivors concerning the mean area of craniectomy (84.7 ± 16.7 cm^2 and 82.8 ± 15.6 cm^2). The mean distance to the skull base was 1.7 ± 1.3 cm and 2.3 ± 1.3 cm ($p = .27$), respectively [28]. In this study we could not demonstrate an influence of the craniectomy size on the outcome. The analysis of the raw data showed that the two main reasons for these results were the wide range of craniectomy sizes and the still too small numbers of patients. Furthermore, this emphasizes the need for further investigations.

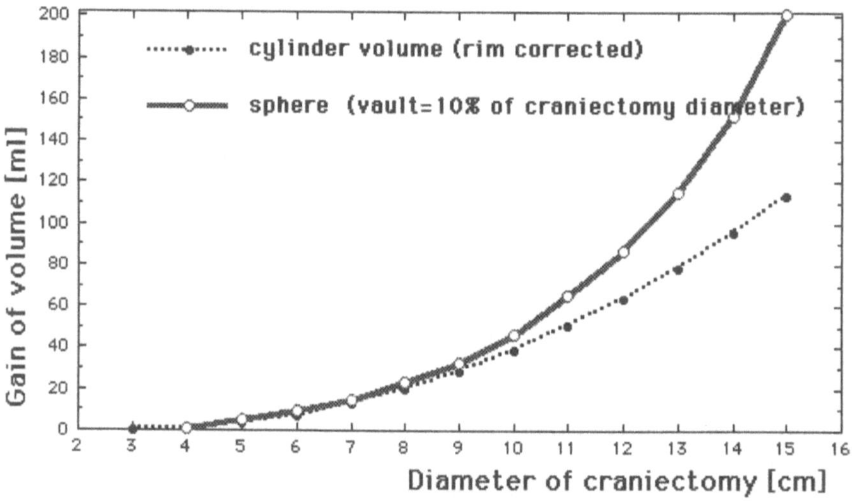

Fig. 6. Mathematical correlation of size craniectomy and volume effect

We had 6 complications. Three epidural, 1 subdural and 2 parenchymal bleeds. One of these was due to an ICP device. Five patients underwent surgical revision and improved with no additional neurological deficit. There were no infections.

Our operation technique consists of removal of a large bone flap, including the frontal, parietal, temporal, and parts of the occipital squama, with consecutive dura plasty (Fig. 7).

Conclusion

Decompressive surgery in patients with malignant MCA infarction improves mortality to less than 30%, compared to 72% in the control group. The majority

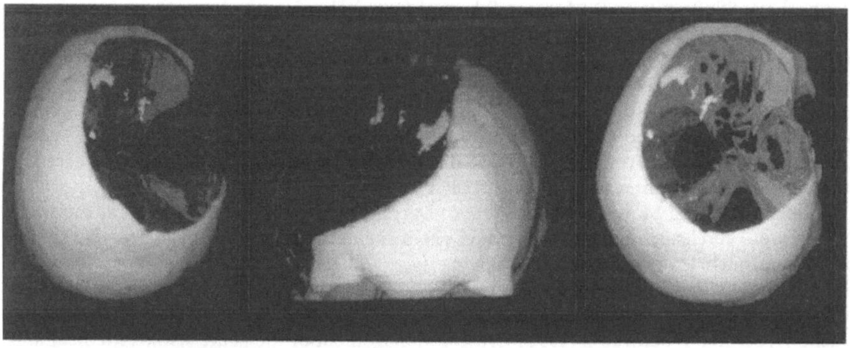

Fig. 7. Three dimensional reconstruction of cCT from 3 views illustrating the extension of the neurosurgical procedure

of surgically treated patients needs little or no help for their activities of daily living and show slightly to moderately severe neurological deficits. This can be regarded as an acceptable functional result.

Timing of craniectomy in patients with malignant MCA infarction is a "dynamic" decision procedure. Patients should be selected carefully for decompressive craniotomy. Craniectomy should be performed after the diagnosis has been confirmed by CCT and if it is not possible to keep CPP above 70 mmHg with conservative treatment. If available, timing of surgery might additionally be supported by $ptiO_2$ and CBF measurements, if these values decrease correlating with an ICP increase. It is probably too late for surgery if pupils are dilated on both sides and do not react to light, indicating irreversible transtentorial herniation.

The diameter of craniectomy should at least be larger than 10 to 12 cm. The bone edges should be smoothly flattened to avoid brain compression at the skull and congestion of cortical veins, which can cause elevation of ICP and intracerebral bleeding. We believe that craniectomy in malignant MCA infarction is a useful therapy and is successful in a well selected patient population.

References

1. Hacke W, Schwab S, Horn M, et al (1996) "Malignant" middle cerebral artery territory infarction. Arch Neurol 53:309–315
2. Shaw CM, Alvord EC, Berry GR (1959) Swelling of the brain following ischemic infarction with arterial occlusion. Arch Neurol 1:161–177
3. Ropper AH, Shafran B (1984) Brain edema after stroke. Clinical syndrome and intracranial pressure. Arch Neurol 41:26–29
4. Ng L, Nimmannitya J (1970) Massive cerebral infarction with severe brain swelling. A clinicopathological study. Stroke 1:158–163
5. Rieke K, Schwab S, Krieger D, et al (1996) Decompressive surgery in space occupying hemispheric infarction: Results of an open, prospective trial. Crit Care Med 23:1576–1587
6. Schwab S, Aschoff A, Spranger M, et al (1996) The value of intracranial pressure monitoring in acute hemispheric stroke. Neurology 47:393–398
7. Ivamoto H, Numoto M, Donaghy R (1974) Surgical decompression for cerebral and cerebellar infarcts. Stroke 5:365–370
8. Rengachary SS, Batnitzky S, Morantz RA, et al (1981) Hemicraniectomy for acute massive cerebral infarction. Neurosurgery 8:321–328
9. Kondziolka D, Fazl M (1988) Functional recovery after decompressive craniectomy for cerebral infarction. J Neurosurg 23:143–147
10. Young PH, Smith KJ, Dunn RC (1982) Surgical decompression after cerebral hemispheric stroke: Indications and patient selection. South Med J 75:473–475
11. Delashaw JB, Broaddus WC, Kassell NF, et al (1990) Treatment of right hemispheric cerebral infarction by hemicraniectomy. Stroke 21:874–881
12. Doerfler A, Forsting M, Reith W, et al (1996) Decompressive craniectomy in a rat model of "malignant" cerebral hemispheric stroke: experimental support for an aggressive therapeutic approach. J Neurosurg 85:853–859
13. Forsting M, Reith W, Schaebitz WR, et al (1995) Decompressive craniectomy for cerebral infarction. An experimental study in rats. Stroke 26:259–264
14. Hacke W, Steiner T, Schwab S (1995) Critical Management of the acute stroke: Medical and Surgical Therapy, in Cerebrovascular Disease, Batjer HH, (Ed). Raven Press Ltd. New York
15. Steiner T, Mendoza G, De Georgia M, et al (1997) Prognosis of stroke patients requiring mechanical ventilation in a neurologic care unit. Stroke 28:711–715

16. Krieger D, Jauss M, Schwarz S et al (1995) Serial somatosensory and brainstem auditory evoked potentials in monitoring of acute supratentorial mass lesions. Crit Care Med 23:1123–1131
17. von Kummer R, Bozzao L, Manelfe C (1994) Early CT diagnosis of hemispheric brain infarction. 1995, Berlin Heidelberg New York Barcelona Budapest Hong Kong London Milan Paris Paris Tokyo, Springer Verlag
18. von Kummer R, Meyding-Lamadé U, Michael F, et al (1994) Sensitivity and prognostic value of early CT in occlusion of the middle cerebral artery trunk. AJNR 15:9–15
19. Forsting M, Krieger D, von Kummer R (1993) The prognostic value of collateral blood flow in acute middle cerebral artery occlusion, in thrombolytic therapy in acute ischemic stroke. del Zoppo GJ, Mori E, Hacke W, (eds) Springer Verlag: Berlin, pp 53–58
20. Saito I, Segawa H, Shiokawa Y, et al (1987) Middle cerebral artery occlusion: Correlation of computed toomgraphy and angiography with clinical outcome. Stroke 18:863–868
21. Smiley G (1952) Occlusive cerebrovascular diseae simulating brain tumor: Angiographic differentiation. Arch Neurol Psychiatr 67:633–640
22. Changaris DG, Mc Graw P, Richardson DJ, et al (1987) Correlation of cerebral perfusion pressure and Glasgow Coma Scale to outcome. J Trauma 27:1007–1013
23. Robertson CS (1983) Treatment of hypertension associated with head injury. J Neurosurg 59:455–460
24. Chan KH, Miller JD, Dearden NM, et al (1992) The effect of changes in cerebral perfusion pressure upon middle cerebral artery blood flow velocity and jugular bulb venous oxygen saturation after severe brain injury. J Neurosurg 77:55–61
25. Rosner MJ, Rosner SD, Johnson AH (1995) Cerebral perfusion pressure: managament protocol and clinical results. J Neurosurg 83:949–962
26. Steiner T, Pilz J, Schellinger P, et al (1997) Continous measurement of tissue oxygen pressure in patients with massive cerebral infarction. Stroke 28:242 (Abst)
27. Keller E, Schwarz S, Bertram M, Schwab S, Hacke W (1997) A new method of bedside-monitoring of Cerebral Blood Flow (CBF) in critical ill patients (Abst). J Cerebrovasc Dis 7:24
28. Wirtz CR, Steiner T, Aschoff A, et al (1997) Hemicraniectomy with dural augmentation in medically uncontrollable hemispheric infarction. Neurosurgical Focus 2:Article 3

Intracerebral Hemorrhage Progression

T. Brott and H. Hennes

Introduction

Bleeding often continues beyond the first hour after intracerebral hemorrhage (ICH), and clinical deterioration is due partly to this continued bleeding. Clinical evaluation is thus far the only means for identifying patients in whom bleeding is continuing, but new tools such as near infra-red spectroscopy (NIRS) may promote early identification of superficial hematomas.

Progression vs Pseudo-Progression of Intracerebral Hemorrhage

During the first 6 hours Fisher hypothesized that expansion of spontaneous intracerebral hemorrhage resulted from a cycle: the initial vessel rupture results in accumulating mass effect, which leads to rupture of immediately surrounding vessels, leading to more mass effect with further and ongoing rupture of surrounding vessels [1]. The mechanisms underlying this expansion were explored in a recent study [2]. Objectives were to determine the percentage of 103 patients with ICH who had evidence of ongoing intracerebral bleeding as measured by serial computed tomography (CT) scans during the first 20 hours after onset of spontaneous ICH, to determine whether continued bleeding was the major cause of early neurologic deterioration, and to explore the possibility of a therapeutic window within the first 24 hours after onset of ICH.

All patients had spontaneous ICH. Patients with cerebral aneurysm, arteriovenous malformations and those taking anticoagulants were excluded. First CT and neurological examination were done within 3 hours of symptom onset. Second CT and neurological examination were done 1 hour after the first examination. Similar evaluations were done at 20 hours and 72 hours after symptom onset. Examination included the Glasgow Coma Scale, the National Institutes of Health (NIH) stroke scale, and metabolic measures. The study was carried out by investigators at each of 12 hospitals. This included a population catchment area of about 1.5 million.

The criterion for hematoma growth was a 10% or greater increase in the radius of the lesion, equivalent to a 33% increase in volume. The average hematoma volume at baseline, 26 cc, is approximately the size of a ping pong ball. At this volume, case mortality at 30 days was 37%. As the lesion increases to about the size of a golf ball, 42 cc, mortality increases to over 70%.

Table 1. Patients with hemorrhage growth >33%

Location	No. cases	Baseline to 1-hour CT		Baseline to 20-hour CT	
		n	%	*n*	%
Putamen	38	10	26	13	34
Thalamic	30	10	33	15	50
Lobar	19	5	26	6	32
Cerebellar	4	0	0	0	0
Pontine	5	1	20	2	40
Other	7	1	14	3	43
Total	103	27	26	39	38

At the baseline to 1 hour CT scan, 26% of the patients had an increase in ICH-volume of more than 33%. An additional 12% of the patients had an increase of 33% or more in ICH-volume. In total, 38% of patients had ongoing bleeding during the first 20 hours after spontaneous ICH. Bleeding risk varied depending on ICH location (Table 1). There were 38 putaminal hemorrhages, of which 26% progressed at 1 hour and 34% at 20 hours after onset.

The growth of ICH was mainly in the acute period, during the first 5 hours. This period is a time of much greater likelihood of clinical change than clinicians are accustomed to seeing with acute ischemic infarction. Neurologists are having more stroke patients referred to as urgent because of available therapies and can expect to see more spontaneous ICH cases who are within this period. A question the investigators were not able to answer was, why does the bleeding stop when it does?

Patients with more than 33% ICH growth had the baseline CT slightly earlier (1.3 vs 1.5 hours from onset) and larger ICH volumes at the 1-hour CT scan. They were also likely to have more than a 2 point drop in GCS and a change in NIH Stroke Scale. However, these patients were not devastated at baseline. Blood pressure did not vary between the two groups with regard to growth versus no growth of the ICH. Thirty-day mortality also did not differ. These data suggest that bleeding in ICH often continues after the first hour, particularly in patients with early clinical deterioration and that clinical deterioration during the first hours after onset is at least partly due to continued bleeding. This is important because patients in this study were broadly representative of ICH patients in the community [3].

Early Detection of Intracerebral Hemorrhage Using Near Infrared Spectroscopy

Time to treatment is the single most important factor in emergency stroke treatment. Early identification of hemorrhagic and ischemic strokes will increase the number of patients who can benefit from interventions. The time frame in treating acute stroke is from 3–6 hours [4, 5]. Near-infrared spectroscopy (NIRS) may help improve the timing of initial diagnosis in stroke and detection of intracranial hematomas because it is particularly sensitive to hemoglobin concentration. This can be used to evaluate differences in optical density between the hemispheres [6]. Optical density will be lower in the side with a hematoma (Fig. 1).

An important consideration for using NIRS is a set of fixed measuring points (Fig. 2). These are used in conjunction with CT scan to find corresponding slices of the CT scan for NIRS measurements (Fig. 3).

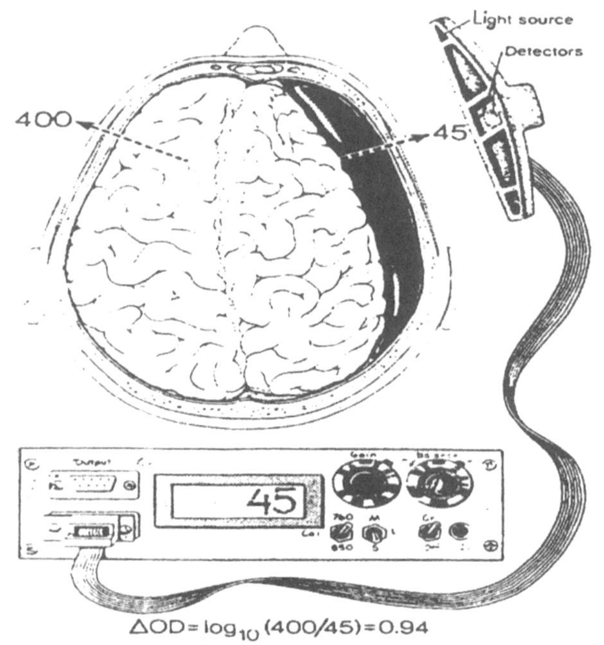

Fig. 1. Differences in optical density between hemispheres

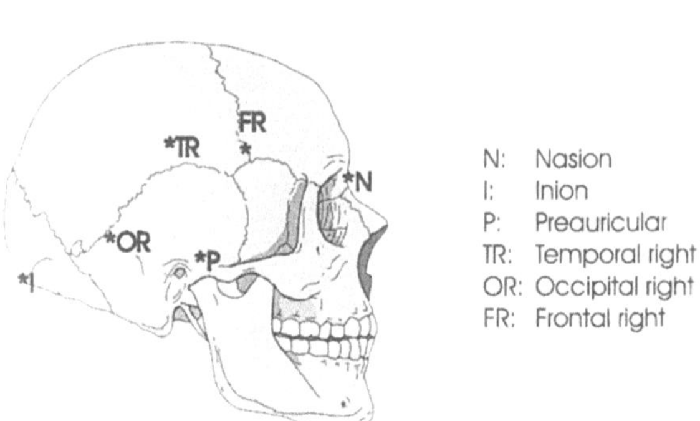

Fig. 2. Measuring points (based on 10/20 system)

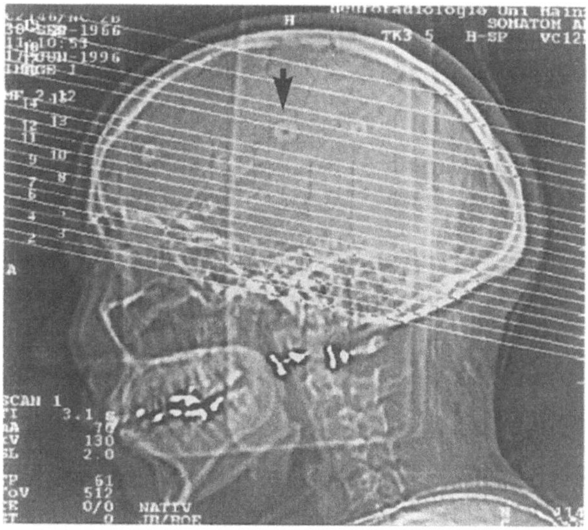

Fig. 3. NIRS diagnostic measuring points

A prospective blinded study of NIRS prior to CT scan was done in 90 patients referred with clinical symptoms of stroke (39 female, 49 male) [7]. Mean age of the first 88 patients was 60.3 (range 16–92) years. Median GCS at presentation was 13.4. Sixteen patients had subdural hematoma, 18 had intraparenchymal hematoma, and 32 had no hemorrhage. Patients with subarachnoid hemorrhage, malignant glioma, galea hematoma, missing CT scans, or who were uncooperative were excluded. The time from obtaining informed consent to the beginning of CT scan was 31.3 minutes (15–50 minutes). NIRS was done at wavelength of 760 nanometers for the detection of hemoglobin.

NIRS sensitivity rate compared to CT scan was 0.8. Specificity was 0.67. If deeper hematomas are excluded, sensitivity rises to 0.9 but specificity remains 0.67.

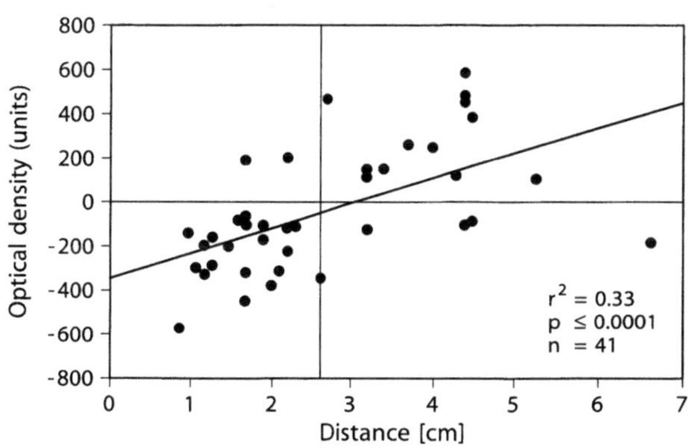

Fig. 4. Depth of hematoma vs. optical density

Plotting depth of the hematoma versus optical density (Fig. 4) shows that for the first 2.5 cm from the skin there is a negative difference in optical density between the hemispheres, with the side which has the hematoma having a lower optical density. This relationship does not hold for deeper hematomas, for unknown reasons. We speculate that NIRS may be confounded by something in the area proximal to the hematoma such as impaired perfusion or edema.

This study showed that NIRS is useful for superficial but not deep hematomas. Measurements are most accurate in hematomas within the first 2.5 cm of depth from the skin surface. Clinical use of NIRS for hematoma detection will require increased depth of light penetration, improved specificity of hematoma detection, and rapid and simplified data collection.

Conclusion

A major goal of intervention in ICH is to stop continued bleeding and growth of the lesion. Studies with serial CT scans show that in 38% of the patients, ICH increases by 33% or more in the first 20 hours after spontaneous hemorrhage. In 26% of the patients that increase occurs within the first hour, and in all patients most of the bleeding is within the first 5 hours. This continued bleeding is at least partly responsible for clinical deterioration during the first 5 hours. Early detection of intracranial hematomas is expected to contribute to improved outcomes. NIRS may be a useful tool for such early detection, at least in superficial hematomas.

References

1. Fisher CM (1971) Pathological observations in hypertensive cerebral hemorrhages. J Neuropathol Exp Neurol 30:536–550
2. Brott T, Broderick J, Kothari R, et al (1997) Early hemorrhage growth in patients with intracerebral hemorrhage. Stroke 28:1–5
3. Broderick J, Brott T, Tomsick T, et al (1994) Management of intracerebral hemorrhage in a large metropolitan population. Neurosurgery 35(5):882–887
4. Hacke W, Kaste M, Fieschi C, et al (1995) Intravenous thrombolysis with recombinant tissue plasminogen activator for acute hemispheric stroke. The European Cooperative Acute Stroke Study. JAMA 274:1017–1025
5. The National Institute of Neurological Disorders and Stroke rt-PA Stroke Study Group (1995) Tissue plasminogen activator for acute ischemic stroke. New Engl J Med 333:1581–1587
6. Gopinath SP, Robertson CS, Grossman RG, et al (1993) Near-infrared spectroscopic localization of intracranial hematomas. J Neurosurgery 79:43–47
7. Hennes HJ, Lott C, Hanley D, et al (1996) Detection of intracranial hematomas using near-infrared spectroscopy (NIRS). J Neurosurg Anesth 8:337–341

Surgical Treatment of Intracerebral Hemorrhage

S. Tuhrim, J. Grotta, H. Hondo, U. Gryzska

Introduction

Treatment of intracerebral hemorrhage (ICH) may include medical management or surgical evacuation. When bleeding is due to an arteriovenous malformation (AVM) treatment may include combined neurosurgical/neuroradiological approaches. Currently there are accepted indications for early evacuation by open craniotomy in some types of ICH. Where indicated, this approach can be expected to reduce mortality, but the effect on functional outcome is less certain. Japanese researchers have pioneered the use of endoscopic evacuation in acute stages, sometimes with local application of thrombolytic agents, but this approach needs to be tested in controlled trials with other modalities. In cases related to arteriovenous malformations, treatment can be improved by a joint neuroradiological/neurosurgical approach.

Operation for Intracerebral Hemorrhage

The main reasons for surgical evacuation of ICH are to decrease mass effect, to improve tissue perfusion, and to prevent accumulation of toxic products. Evacuation of ICH is now thought to be definitely indicated for cerebellar hemorrhage with brainstem compression or hemorrhage secondary to another lesion requiring surgery. Less definite indications include putamenal or lobar hemorrhage with decreased level of consciousness or progressive deterioration. Possible indications include any putamenal or thalamic hemorrhage greater than 30 cc as well as smaller thalamic or pontine hemorrhages that can be evacuated via stereotactic aspiration.

Current practice of patient selection for surgical vs medical therapy is not based on results of randomized clinical trials. The chosen modality is primarily based on personal clinical experience, local surgical custom, and the resources available. Consequently, surgical rates vary geographically from over 50% in Japan to under 20% in the US.

There is still controversy about the management of intracerebral hemorrhage. Beginning with McKissock et al., most randomized trials have observed no benefit from surgery [1]. However, Auer et al. showed benefits from surgical treatment in a study of endoscopic removal of supratentorial hemorrhages. Patients with subcortical hematomas had a significantly lower mortality rate (30% vs 70%) and the survivors had better outcomes than those treated medically [2]. A formal statistical meta-analysis of all randomized trials of medical therapy versus surgical therapy shows no difference between the two, but when analysis is confined to series following the introduction of computed tomography (CT), surgery appears beneficial in reducing mortality [3].

The main decision-making criteria in most clinics appear to be the patient's clinical condition, the site and size of the hematoma, the underlying pathology, and timing. The etiology is usually hypertensive but may have other causes which can affect the decision about surgery. The most common causes of ICH are hypertension, arteriovenous malformation (AVM), aneurysm, tumor, amyloid angiopathy, chronic encapsulated hematoma, and bleeding diatheses including clotting disorders, thrombocytopenia, anticoagulation, and thrombolysis. A number of attempts have been made at multivariate modeling. These generally agree that the size of the hemorrhage, the Glasgow Coma Scale score or level of consciousness, and whether or not there is blood in the ventricular system are highly predictive of outcome [4]. However, these are not necessarily predictive of whether surgery is likely to be of benefit.

AVM or aneurysm may dictate a particular surgical approach, as will be explained later. Tumor usually requires surgery. There is controversy over whether amyloid angiopathy presents a greater surgical challenge. Chronic encapsulated hematoma may require surgery if it is behaving like a tumor. Bleeding diatheses suggest a problem with hemostasis and may affect prognosis, particularly in the short term.

The location of the hematoma is of major importance, although there are as yet no reliable multivariate models in regard to infratentorial locations. Brainstem pontine hematomas can be operated but this is currently the exception rather than the rule. There is a suggestion that with microsurgical techniques or aspiration moderate-sized hematomas may benefit from removal, but certainly there are no predictive models that permit conclusions one way or the other.

Rules of thumb have been developed with cerebellar hematoma. Cerebellar hematoma accounts for 10% of ICH (Table 1). The critical size for surgical treatment is 3 cm diameter. Clinical criteria for surgery include impairment of consciousness or other signs of brainstem compression, with or without the develop-

Table 1. Allocation of intracerebral hemorrhages

Location	All intracerebral hemorrhages (%)
Cerebellar	10
Brainstem	10
Thalamus	15
Putamen	35
Lobar	25
Other	5

ment of obstructive hydrocephalus. Surgery done before the patient becomes stuporous or comatose has a 75% survival rate. Surgery after that point has a 75% mortality rate [5].

Brainstem hematomas account for 10% of ICH, and 85% of these are pontine. They are usually treated medically. Microsurgical decompression or stereotactic aspiration can be beneficial in moderate size (5–10 cc) hematomas.

Fifteen percent of ICH occur in the thalamus. Such hematomas are usually not evacuated. Ventricular drainage for intraventricular hemorrhage (IVH) that accompanies thalamic hemorrhage may be beneficial, but this has not proven in controlled trials. Stereotactic aspiration may be beneficial but also has not been proven.

The most common site for ICH is the putamen, which accounts for about 35% of such occurrences. Indications for evacuation are impairment of consciousness or a size greater than 30 cc. Patients with diminished level of consciousness are the most likely to benefit from surgery [6].

About 25% of ICH are lobar, and these are of more diverse etiologies than hemorrhages in other sites. Temporal lobe ICH may be more likely to herniate and may thus have worse outcomes [7]. Patients with such lesions may be more likely to benefit from surgery. Those with moderate size (30–80 cc) hemorrhages are also more likely to benefit from evacuation.

One problem with attempts to develop a multivariate model thus far is that few of the patients in these studies were seen within 6 or even 12 hours of onset. Hemorrhages can expand within the first several hours, perhaps even up to the first 6 hours [8,9]. In noncomatose patients 1/3 evaluated early subsequently deteriorated [10]. In patients evaluated within 3 hours of onset, the early volume of ICH but not the Glasgow Coma Scale score predicted outcome, at least among patients conscious at evaluation [11].

As patients are evaluated earlier in the clinical setting, predictive models will have to be revised. Hardemark et al. reported that hematoma evacuation might decrease early mortality in patients with GCS under 6 and hematoma volume under 60 mL. Hardemark also reported that evacuation seems to be harmful in patients with smaller hematomas [12]. However, in patients evaluated within 12 hours of onset, none of the variables including size of hematoma predicted outcome in those who were operated vs those who were not.

An example of the unreliability of current models is the case report of a 45 year-old man seen within an hour of onset. He was slightly lethargic but otherwise had relatively good cognitive status and GCS. He had normal pulse pressure when initially evaluated, along with a major hematoma of about 80 cc. (Fig. 1a–e).

We would have predicted that he would survive, probably with a good outcome at one year, but by the time he returned to the emergency room after the CT scan his pulse pressure had gone up, his GCS was now 8, and he had an increased probability of death or poor outcome. This demonstrates that the timing of when one evaluates the patient may be crucial in terms of deciding which predictive models and predictors are useful.

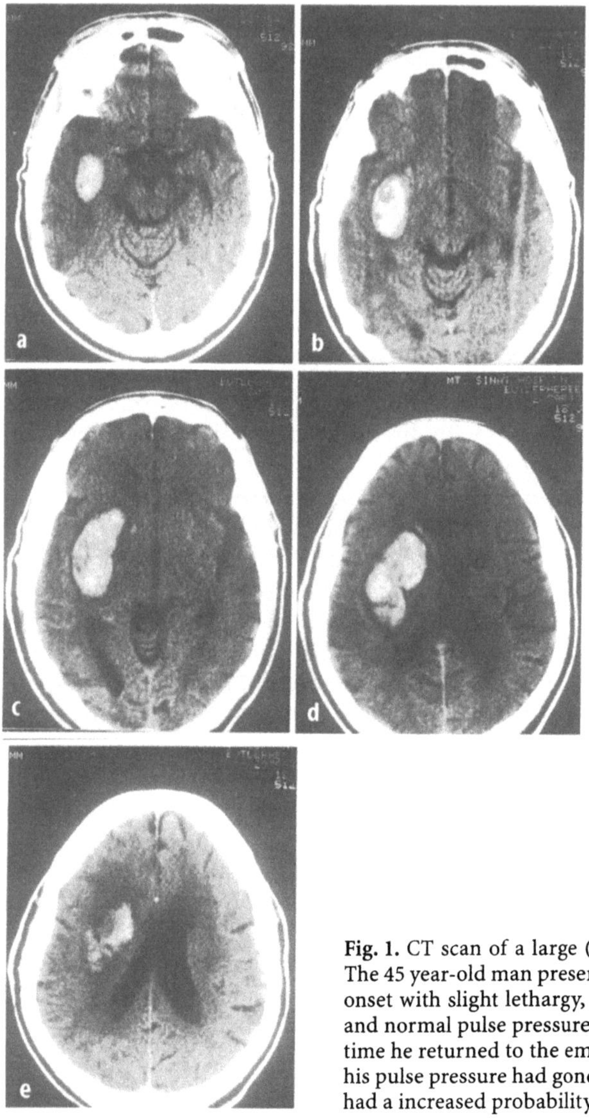

Fig. 1. CT scan of a large (80 cc) intracerebral hematoma. The 45 year-old man presented within an hour of symptom onset with slight lethargy, good cognitive status and GCS, and normal pulse pressure when initially evaluated. By the time he returned to the emergency room after the CT scan his pulse pressure had gone up, his GCS score was 8, and he had a increased probability of death or poor outcome

Controlled Trial in Spontaneous Ganglionic ICH

Broderick et al. previously compared patients undergoing surgery with deep or lobar hemorrhage with those not undergoing operation (Table 2). They found that 29 of 157 patients received surgery and that operated patients tended to be younger and to have lobar hematomas. Glasgow Coma Scales were about the same for operated vs not operated patients, but hematomas were slightly larger in the surgical group. There was a trend toward lower mortality in patients who

Table 2. Patients with deep or lobar hemorrhage treated with of without surgery

Variable	Operation ($n=29$)	No operation ($n=128$)	P
Mean time from onset to first medical evaluation (hr)	5±14	3±5	0.54
Age (yr)	58±17	72±15	0.0001
Initial Glasgow Coma Scale Score	11±3	11±3	0.43
Volume of ICH (mL)	50±31	37±38	0.10
Lobar location (%)	64	43	0.05
30-day mortality (%)	25	46	0.06
Modified Oxford Handicap Scale Score	4.7±1.2	4.6±1.7	0.77

were operated, but no difference in functional outcomes as measured by the modified Oxford Handicap Scale scores [13].

Juvela et al. reported a randomized study of open craniotomy vs medical management in 52 patients. They found a worse outcome in the surgical group [14]. In open craniotomy done after computed tomography became available, there are no randomized prospective data showing that surgery is beneficial.

One such trial is now in the planning stages. The Surgical Treatment of Intracerebral Hemorrhage (STICH) study objectives are: (1) to determine if early hematoma evacuation improves survival from ICH; (2) to determine if early hematoma evacuation improves functional outcome in survivors from ICH; and (3) to determine which ICH subtypes benefit most from surgery. The study is being conducted by Lewis B. Morgenstern, William Pasteur, Peter Shedden, James C. Grotta, and the University of Texas at Houston Stroke Team.

The most important inclusion criterion is supratentorial ICH larger than 10 cc by CT scan. We have found that because hematomas continue to enlarge, many patients first seen with intracerebral hemorrhages greater than 10 cc still have bad outcomes. Putamenal and lobar hematomas 10 cc or smaller nearly always do well. Since the goal of the study is to look at patients in the early phases of ICH, we decided to err on the side of smaller volume.

The study also requires randomization and surgery within 4 hours of symptom onset and initial Glasgow Coma Scale scores of 5–15. Wide awake patients are included because some such patients present at the emergency room in the first few hours and then ultimately die of edema and enlargement of the hematoma. Patients must be over age 17, and of course informed consent must be obtained.

Exclusion criteria include ICH secondary to AVM, aneurysm, brain tumor, or head trauma. Patients are also excluded if intraventricular bleeding occupies greater than half of both lateral ventricles or over 2/3 of one lateral ventricle. It is difficult to measure volume in such lesions, and patients often have drainage of blood through a ventriculostomy, which would make data difficult to analyze. Patients are also excluded if they have low function prior to ICH (Rankin >2), coagulopathy or serious surgical risk factors.

The volume of hematoma is calculated by measuring the slice showing the largest cross-sectional area of hematoma. Since most hematomas are ellipsoid, volume can be calculated by multiplying the largest diameter by the perpendicular diameter, multiply that by the number of slices and thickness of slices (5 mm or 10 mm), and dividing the final number by 2.

Results of the pilot study for this trial include 11 patients randomized to surgery and 15 to medical treatment within 12 hours of hematoma onset. Their average GCS score was 11, and average hematoma volume was 50–60 cc. Mortality was 9% with surgical evacuation and 27% with medical treatment. The preliminary data suggest that open craniotomy does seem to be improving mortality in these patients. Barthel scores at 30 days after treatment were 17.7 with surgery vs 23.7 with medical therapy. It is clear that outcome is poor with either medical therapy or surgery delayed 12 hours. Because of the high incidence of hematoma enlargement over the first few hours and the effects of blood on the brain, researchers have shortened the time window for surgery in future studies to four hours.

Patients who refused randomization are being followed prospectively. Fourteen have been treated with surgery and 16 with medical therapy. Mortality of the patients who refused randomization was 22% with surgery and 39% with medical treatment. Barthel scores 30 days after treatment were 16 with surgery and 29 with medical therapy.

Later Barthel scores found substantial improvement in the surgically treated patients between 30 days and 6 months, reflecting the fact that recovery from hematomas is slower than after infarctions. Barthel scores suggest that it is not realistic to think of curing patients with large hematomas by surgical evacuation, but mortality and severe disability may be improved with prompt surgical treatment. Early surgery may reduce mortality from ICH, but these data suggest that it does not dramatically improve functional outcomes in survivors. However, it remains possible that surgical evacuation may decrease the number of patients left severely disabled. A multi center study is needed to confirm these results, to determine whether new surgical techniques such as endoscopic or stereotactic surgery are more beneficial than open craniotomy, to determine which subgroups (e.g. lobar vs putamenal ICH) benefit most from surgery, and to determine which medical techniques (e.g. blood pressure management) improve or worsen functional outcome.

A number of unanswered questions remain: What is the minimal amount of ICH which should be included for a surgical evacuation trial? Which surgical approach (open craniotomy, stereotactic aspiration, or endoscopic removal) should be used in which circumstances? What situations call for instillation of thrombolytics?

A further need is for standardization of the criteria for monitoring intracranial pressure (ICP). All of the critical care management of these patients would benefit from standardization to permit comparison of results across multiple centers.

The research setting raises some particular concerns. In clinical trials, should there be crossover from medical to surgical management of a patient who is randomized to medical management and then deteriorates? There are as yet no good data indicating that such delayed surgery is useful.

Clinically, questions arise about what constitutes successful clot evacuation. Many patients have residual blood if re-scanned after surgical evacuation. Studies are needed to determine whether residual blood correlates with success of surgery.

Cerebral blood flow studies show substantial hypoperfusion around hematomas, along with the center core of very severe reduction of blood flow that corresponds to the volume of the hematoma. Edema and ischemic problems occurring in concert with the hematoma are likely to be important targets for future therapies.

Endoscopic and Stereotactic Evacuation

Histological changes around a hematoma following intracerebral hemorrhage begin with 6–7 hours and reach a maximum 3–4 days after onset [15]. Evacuating the hematoma in the acute stage may help limit damage. Ultrasonic aspiration can break up clots and help evacuate hematomas in the acute stage. This suggests that histological change can be limited by evacuating the hematoma in the acute stage.

Endoscopic surgery can be used when the clinician needs to aspirate the hard clot in the acute stage. (Aspiration of chronic hematoma is easier because typically the clot is partly dissolved.) Various mechanical devices have been tried in attempts to improve clot removal. These include the Archimedes screw, a coaxial double cannula, and the ultrasonic aspirator and water jet [16–18]. With this device a stream of water comes down and breaks up the hematoma, which is then aspirated.

In some cases, aspiration may be a viable alternative to open craniotomy for evacuation of ICH. Stereotactic aspiration surgery is less invasive than open surgery and can be carried out under local anesthesia. Operative time is brief. The apparatus is relatively simple. Deep-seated hematomas, and thalamic or pontine hemorrhage can also be aspirated using this method. It may also be appropriate for elderly or high-risk patients. Endoscopic aspiration is not indicated for patients with expanding hematomas.

Ultrasound, fibrinolysis, and lasers have been used to break up the clot and facilitate endoscopic aspiration. Using ultrasound, the hematoma is fragmented at the end of a cannula, through which it is then aspirated. In many cases nearly total evacuation of the hematoma can be carried out (Fig. 2). However, to avoid intraoperative bleeding the volume of hematoma aspirated should be limited to about 70% of the estimated hematoma.

Fibrinolysis of hematoma has been reported by several authors [19]. We have reported experience with 51 patients who had undergone manual aspiration through a silicone tube of 3.5 mm o.d. this was followed by administration of urokinase, aspiration, and further injection of urokinase every 6–12 hours until the clot was totally removed. The hematoma usually disappeared 2 or 3 days postoperatively [20].

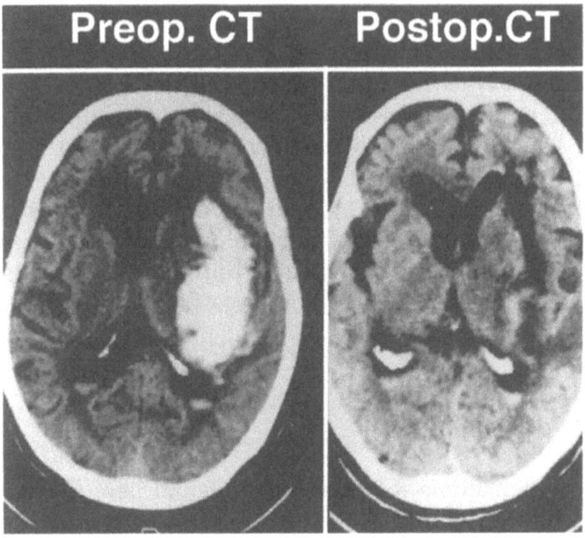

Fig. 2. Endoscopic evacuation of hematoma (from: Ebina K, Brain Hemorrhage '95, 1995)

Using endoscopic evacuation, the hematoma can be evacuated under visual observation, and the bleeding point can be coagulated by laser or electrocoagulator. In this approach, a small burr hole is made, the edge of the burr hole is widened to facilitate probe insertion, and the patient is transferred to the CT room. The head is immobilized, the probe is set, and the tip is placed on the cortex. CT images are taken. The target point is determined at the center of the hematoma, and the x and y values of the coordinates are obtained by the cursor number of the CT scan. Coordinates of the burr hole point are obtained by the same method. Direction of the fixed probe is confirmed by coordinates of an N1 slice, which is located at the same point as the burr hole, and N2 slice which is located distal to the N1 position of the probe. The crossing point of the x and y axes indicates a predetermined target point. After confirmation of the direction of the fixed probe, the probe is inserted to the predetermined point. The tip of the needle is checked by CT scan. Aspiration of the hematoma is done by the ultrasonic hematoma aspirator and confirmed by postoperative CT scan.

Positioning the needle for aspiration can be done using ultrasound-guided, CT-guided (with or without frame) or MRI-guided stereotaxy. The CT-guided method is most common (Fig. 3). Stereotactic aspiration can be used for putamenal, thalamic, cerebellar, pontine, and subcortical hemorrhages. Use is determined by hematoma location, hematoma size, and patient characteristics. Aspiration surgery is recommended for thalamic hemorrhage patients who are alert, stuporous, or semiconscious, with hematoma volume more than 30 mL.

Auer reported a randomized trial of endoscopic surgery vs medical treatment for hypertensive intracerebral hemorrhage [2]. Patients with subcortical hemorrhage had significantly lower mortality and better function after surgical aspiration than did control subjects treated with medical therapy.

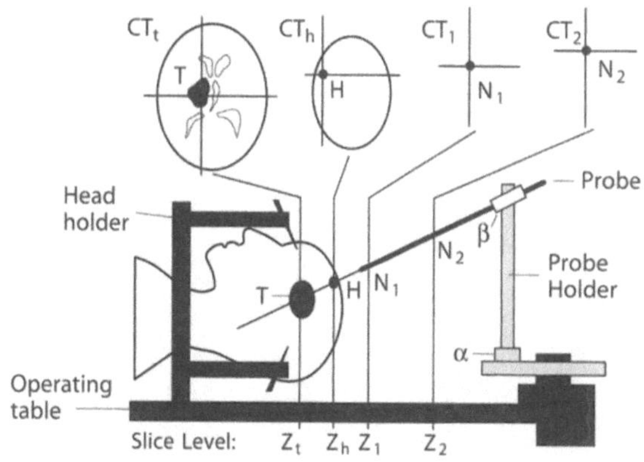

Fig. 3. Stereotactic placement for ultrasonic evacuation of HIH

Intraoperative bleeding is the most serious complication in aspiration surgery for intracerebral hemorrhage. The rebleeding rate differs depending on the method used. The rebleeding rate with manual aspiration is about 4% [21]. Kandel reported a rather high rate of 16% with a motor-driven Archimedes screw [22]. Ultrasonic aspiration method seems to be safe, with a rebleeding rate of 1.6% [23].

Figure 4 illustrates a case of intraoperative bleeding. The perioperative CT shows a putamenal hemorrhage. After the second aspiration systolic blood pressure abruptly increased to 220 mmHg and the CT scan revealed a larger hematoma. Systolic blood pressure was immediately decreased to 100 mmHg and intra-

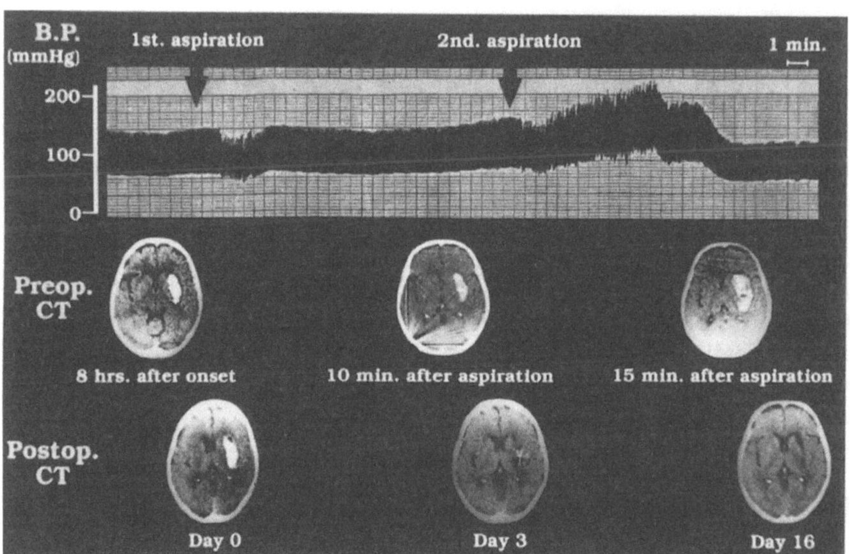

Fig. 4. Rebleeding after aspiration surgery

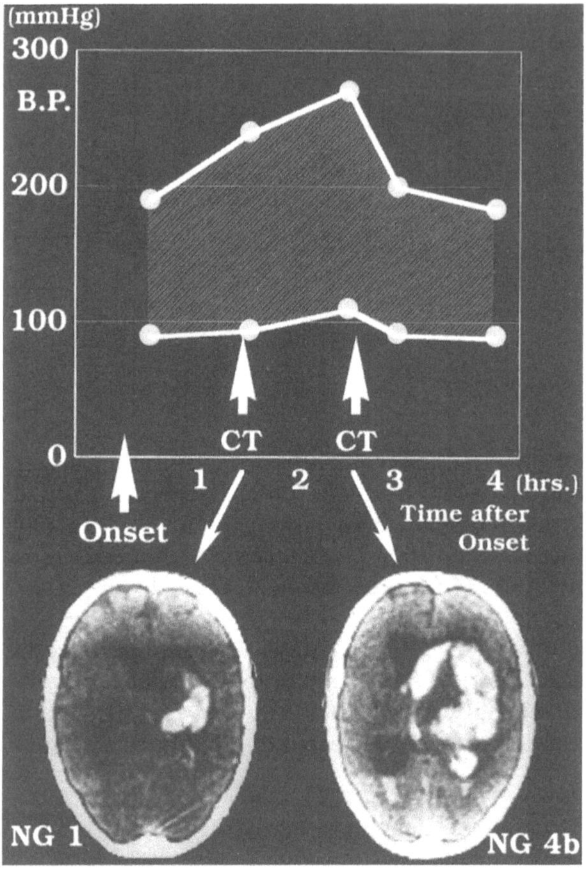

Fig. 5. Hematoma expansion in patients with poor blood pressure control

operative bleeding stopped. The hematoma was drained by urokinase infusion three days after the aspiration. Fortunately this patient did well with urokinase infusion and drainage of the hematoma.

Aspiration should be done no sooner than 6 hours after onset. To avoid intraoperative bleeding, not more than 70% of the clot volume should be aspirated. If intraoperative bleeding occurs, the cannula should be left in place until the bleeding stops, then the blood pressure should be immediately decreased. If the bleeding does not stop, endoscopic coagulation or open surgery are recommended.

Combined Neurosurgical/Neuroradiological Treatment of AVMS

Cerebral arteriovenous malformations (AVMs) carry a high risk of hemorrhage. Combined treatment with embolization, surgery, and radiotherapy can improve outcomes and permit curative treatment of previously intractable lesions. Published reports of 2799 patients treated with surgery alone have an overall 11.8% morbidity and 5.6% mortality [24].

The aim of therapy is complete exclusion of the AVM from the circulation without neurological deficits. Advantages of a combined neurosurgical/neuroradiological approach include advantages of combination treatment increasing number of potentially curable cases; improving medical, social, and economic prognosis; facilitating surgery; reducing the need for transfusions; and reducing the need for postoperative intensive care and rehabilitation. The task for the interventional neuroradiologist is to occlude the nidus and surgically inaccessible feeders, and to eliminate coincidental arteriovenous fistulae and flow-related aneurysms. However, the neuroradiology intervention must not prolong the total treatment procedure in an overzealous effort to reach feeding vessels that are easily accessible for the neurosurgeon. Careful planning should allocate each region of the individual AVM to the appropriate discipline.

Embolization can be used as a preoperative measure to occlude the nidus (preferable via surgically inaccessible feeding vessels), occlude AV fistulas, and occlude distal flow-related aneurysms. However, analysis of the results of AVM embolization showed that a definite cure of an AVM by means of embolization as the only measure is feasible in only 7% of cases. Various materials have been developed for embolization, including Ethibloc emulsion, platinum coils, and PVA particles. Ethibloc is an emulsion of maize prolamine and oleum papaveris, water-soluble contrast medium, and alcohol. It solidifies by means of precipitation after the alcohol has been diluted. This leaves a soft, rubbery occluded vessel which is easier to dissect and manipulate during surgery than the rigid vessels embolized with other materials. PVA particles are used in order to occlude small accessory vessels or perforating arteries. Platinum coils are used to occlude feeders directly behind the angioma in order to embolize it. The preoperative embolization should reduce the time required for surgery, so that the total time required for both procedures would be close to the time needed for surgery of a high-grade angioma.

In a series of 179 consecutive patients with cerebral AVMs has been treated since 1988 at the University Hospital of Hamburg through a system of joint neuroradiological-neurosurgical management. These include 39 patients treated by surgery alone, 6 by embolization alone, and 120 by surgery after embolization. Three were referred for radiotherapy after reduction of angioma size by embolization, 2 received primary radiotherapy only, and 14 were considered to be untreatable.

Results of the combined approaches were promising. Of the 165 patients treated with surgery, embolization, or embolization followed by surgery, 84% were cured (total resection of the angioma without neurologic deficit), 5% had reduced AVMs, 9% had AVMs removed but with some neurological deficit, and 2% died. This is substantially below the 5.6% mortality seen in published series of patients treated with surgery alone, as mentioned before. Among the 19 patients treated with embolization plus radiotherapy, radiotherapy alone, or no therapy, there were no cures, but 16% had reduced AVMs.

Combined neuroradiological and neurosurgical treatment provides the opportunity to operate on even large and complicated malformations safely. Short treatment intervals between radiologic and surgical treatment reduce the risk of secondary arterialization without adversely affecting the operability due to brain edema or other problems. This approach can reduce the overall hospitalization time.

Conclusion

Many questions remain about operative management of ICH, particularly concerning the issues of when surgical evacuation is likely to produce a better outcome than medical therapy. This area requires further research in randomized, controlled clinical trials. Among the questions are when open craniotomy is indicated, and when equal or better results could be obtained by endoscopic evacuation. The use of fibrinolysis, particularly by agents such as urokinase or rtPA, offers the possibility of removing residual clot not evacuated in the initial surgical approach, but this raises a new question: how much of the hematoma should be removed? As neurosurgical and neuroradiological techniques continue to evolve, joint neurosurgical/neuroradiological management of cases should become more common.

References

1. McKissock W, Richardson A, Taylor J (1961) Primary intracerebral hemorrhage. A controlled trial of surgical and conservative treatment in 180 unselected cases. Lancet 2:221–236
2. Auer LM, Deinsberger W, Niederkorn K, et al (1989) Endoscopic surgery versus medical treatment for spontaneous intracerebral hematoma: A randomized study. J Neurosurg 70:530–535
3. Saver JL (1994) Surgical therapy. In Feldmann E (ed) Intracerebral Hemorrhage Armonk, NY: Futura Publishing Co., pp 305–306
4. Tuhrim S, Horowitz DR, Sacher H, et al (1995) Validation and comparison of models predicting intracerebral hemorrhage survival. Critical Care Medicine 23:950–954
5. Ott KH, Kane CS, Ojemann RG, Mohr JP (1974) Cerebellar hemorrhage: diagnosis and treatment. A review of 56 cases. Arch Neurol 31:160–167
6. Kanno T, Nagata J, Nonomura K, et al (1992) Treatment of hypertensive intracerebral hemorrhage: new approaches. Eighteenth Princeton Conference, Rochester Hills, MI, 1992
7. Andrews BT, Chiles BW, Olsen WL, et al (1988) The effect of intracerebral hemorrhage location on the risk of brainstem compression and on clinical outcome. J Neurosurg 69:518–522
8. Broderick JP, Brott TG, Tomsick T, et al (1990) Ultra-early evaluation of intracerebral hemorrhage. J Neurosurg 72:195–199
9. Fumitsu K, Muramoto M, Iheda Y, et al (1990) Indications for surgical treatment of putaminal hemorrhage. J Neurosurg 73:518–525
10. Lisk DR, Pasteur W, Rhoades H et al (1994) Early presentation of hemispheric intracerebral hemorrhage: prediction of outcome and guidelines for treatment allocation. Neurology 44:133–139
11. Lippitz BE, Mayfrank L, Spetzger U, et al (1994) Lysis of basal ganglia hematoma with recombinant tissue plasminogen activator (rtPA) after stereotactic aspiration: initial results. Acta Neurochir 127:157–160

12. Hardemark HG, Schwarz S, Wesslen N, et al. Factors associated with early mortality after supratentorial intracerebral hemorrhage. Abstract #9, presented at the Emergency Management and Critical Care of Stroke meeting, Heidelberg, 5-7 September 1996
13. Broderick J, Brott T, Tomsick T, et al (1994) Management of intracerebral hemorrhage in a large metropolitan population. Neurosurgery 34:882–887
14. Juvela S (1996) Prevalence of risk factors in spontaneous intracerebral hemorrhage and aneurysmal subarachnoid hemorrhage. Archives of Neurology 53:734–740
15. Ebina T, Sakurai Y, Suzuki J (1977) Progressive changes of the brain tissue around the experimental hematoma. In: Surgery of Hypertensive Intracerebral Hematoma, Kitamura K (ed) Neuron publishing Co, Tokyo, pp 87–92 (in Japanese)
16. Backlund EO, von Holst H (1978) Controlled subtotal evacuation of intracerebral hematomas by stereotactic technique. Surg Neurol 9:99–101
17. Matsumoto K, Hondo H, Tomida K (1988) Aspiration surgery for hypertensive brain hemorrhage in the acute stage. In: Suzuki J (ed) Advances in Surgery for Cerebral Stroke. Springer-Verlag, Tokyo, pp 433–441
18. Ito H, Mukai H, Kitamura A, et al (1989) Stereotactic aqua stream and aspirator for hypertensive intracerebral hematoma. Stereotac Funct Neurosurg 53:77–84
19. Schaller C, Rhode V, Meyer B, et al (1995) Stereotactic puncture and lysis of spontaneous intracerebral hemorrhage using recombinant tissue-plaminogen activator Neurosurgery 36:328–335
20. Hondo H (1983) CT guided stereotactic evacuation of hypertensive intracerebral hematomas. Tokushima J Exp Med 30:25–39
21. Matsumoto K, hondo H (1984) CT-guided stereotaxic evacuation of hypertensive intracerebral hematomas. J Neurosurg 61:440–448
22. Kandel EI, Peresdov VV (1985) Stereotaxic evacuation of spontaneous intracerebral hematomas. J Neurosurg 62:206–213
23. Hondo H (in press) Perioperative blood pressure management of patients with hypertensive intracerebral hemorrhage in the acute stage. Jpn J Stroke (in Japanese)
24. Gryzska U, Westphal M, Zauella F, et al (1993) A joint protocol for the neurosurgical and neuroradiologic treatment of cerebral arteriovenous malformations: indications, technique, and results in 76 cases. Surg Neurol 40:476–484

Operative and Interventional Neuroradiology

M. Shibuya, R. Higashida, and D. Kühne

Introduction

Endovascular surgery is suitable for both large and giant aneurysms, although additional long-term studies are needed. Use of coils to occlude aneurysms is becoming standard therapy. Endovascular treatment may allow occlusion of aneurysms with little brain trauma and without craniotomy or surgical vessel preparation. Factors that contribute to a good outcome following subarachnoid hemorrhage (SAH) include successful repair of the primary bleeding site, early clot removal, prevention of vasospasm, and prevention of rebleeding. Treatment approaches include both surgical and endovascular modalities.

The incidence of cerebral aneurysms is 1.5–8%, meaning that about 5 million people in North America have intracerebral aneurysms. Aneurysms cause 80,000 acute hemorrhages per year in this population, with a 36% mortality rate and 15–30% stroke rate. The most common symptoms of SAH are shown in Table 1.

Surgical Strategies for Treating Aneurysms and SAH

M. Shibuya

Treatment strategy is determined by whether the aneurysm is ruptured or not. Surgery may be early or delayed, depending on the patient's condition (Fig. 1).

Table 1. Symptoms of subarachnoid hemorrhage

Symptom	Patients (%)
Headache	85
Nausea	44
Vomiting	34
Brief loss of consciousness	32
Neck stiffness or pain	15
Hemiparesis	15
Vertigo	12
Faintness	12
Confusion	7

Adapted from Adams HP et al, JAMA 1980; 244:794

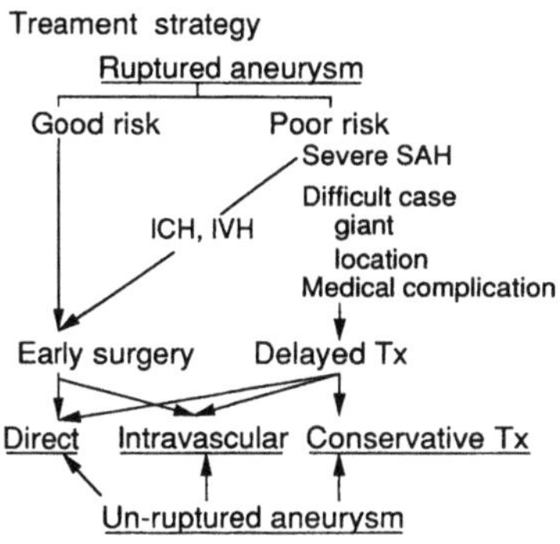

Fig. 1. Aneurysm treatment strategy

Early surgery is defined as that done within 3 days after SAH but before development of vasospasm. In this situation aggressive treatment to prevent or relieve vasospasm can be undertaken. Late surgery is that surgery done 8–12 days after SAH. Timing of delayed surgery may depend on the amount of subarachnoid clot present. Smaller clot permits earlier surgery. This is usually desirable, but the brain is still swollen in early stages compared with later and this may be an important consideration in some cases.

A major international cooperative study of timing concluded that early surgery is advantageous for alert patients but not significantly better than delayed surgery for patients who are stuporous or comatose. The 3,500 patients included 83% who were operated on and 50% in whom surgery was within 3 days after SAH [1]. Kassell et al found that the most favorable results were for alert patients who were operated on within 3 days of SAH. The worst results were with surgery after 7 days. There was little difference in the groups operated on between days 4–6 vs between days 7–14. Rebleeding occurred in 5.7% of patients operated on by day 3, 9.4% of patients operated on during days 4–6, 13.9% of patients operated on during days 7–14, and 21.5% of patients operated on during days 15–32. Mortality ranged from 4% in patients operated on by day 3 to 15.1% in patients operated on during days 15–32. Patients who were stuporous or comatose had similar outcomes regardless of the timing of surgery.

Many neurosurgical centers have moved their aneurysm treatment practices towards early surgery with a strong emphasis on accomplishing successful repair of the primary bleeding site. The outcome of patient series is of interest. Ohman and Heiskanen studied the timing of operation after aneurysmal SAH in 216 patients with a ruptured aneurysm of the anterior part of the circle of Willis. The study included only patients in Hunt and Hess clinical Grades I to III, Patients were admitted and randomly assigned to a treatment group within 72 hours after SAH. Patients were randomly assigned to acute surgery (0 to 3 days after SAH), intermediate surgery (4 to 7 days after SAH), or late surgery (8 days to an indefinite time after SAH). At 3 months post-SAH, 65 patients (91.5%) from the early surgery group were classified as independent compared to 55 (78.6%) from the intermediate surgery group and 56 (80.0%) from the late surgery group [2].

Shibuya has reported a study of 992 patients with SAH treated in 20 hospitals in Japan [3]. Surgery was on day 0–1 in 72% of patients, and by day 3 in 82% of patients. Daily activity at one month after hemorrhage was graded by the Glasgow Outcome Scale. This showed that 57% of patients had returned to their previous activities. Furthermore, 70% were able to live independently. There was 19% morbidity and 11% mortality.

Outcomes correlated with SAH severity. About 86% of Hunt grade 1 or 2 patients were independent at 1 month after SAH, compared to 60% of grade 3 patients and 30% of grade 4 patients. There was also a correlation between outcome and the size of the clot on computed tomography (CT) scan. There was no correlation between outcome and the timing of the aneurysm surgery. Main causes of poor outcome (neurological deficits) were vasospasm (20%), hemorrhage (original or rebleed, 7%), infarction or subdural effusion (6%), surgical complications (5%), and hydrocephalus (4%).

Because vasospasm is the most common cause of poor outcome it has been studied in detail. About 70% of patients had postoperative angiography. Fifty-two percent of these patients showed some angiographic evidence of vasospasm, and 43% showed either transient or permanent neurological deficits due to vasospasm. There was a correlation between the location of the aneurysm and angiographic spasm. Aneurysms in the posterior fossa showed less angiographic spasm than supratentorial aneurysm (7% vs 30%). A similar correlation was found for symptomatic spasm, which occurred in 16% of patients with vertebrobasilar aneurysms but in 50% of patients with anterior cerebral artery aneurysms. These data seem to recommend early surgery, at least for good-grade patients.

There was also a correlation between vasospasm and age for symptomatic vasospasm. It should be noted that we found no association between age and occurrence of angiographic spasm. Thus, older patients have an increased incidence of symptomatic spasm, although their rate of angiographic vasospasm was unchanged. This suggests that older patients show symptoms with less severe angiographic vasospasm.

Vasospasm is caused by the presence of clot in the subarachnoid space. Tsuji et al showed in animal studies that removing the clot within 48 hours prevents vasospasm [4]. A North American cooperative study showed that intraoperative cisternal tPA causes 56% reduction in the risk of severe vasospasm in patients with SAH [5]. A useful technical adjunct to the intracisternal use of tPA is head shaking and cisternal drainage [6].

Rebleeding remains an important cause of poor outcome. The risk of rebleeding is greatest during the first day after SAH [1]. Fujii showed recently that among 179 patients admitted within 24 hours after hemorrhage, 17% rebled, most within 6 hours after the first bleeding [7]. Rebleeding markedly lowers the prospect of a good outcome. They have reported good recovery in 51% of patients who did not have rebleeding but in only 16% of those who did rebleed. Mortality was 18% without rebleeding vs 65% with rebleeding. This suggests that significant morbidity and mortality could be prevented by early surgery and aggressive treatment to prevent development of vasospasm.

Interventional Neuroradiology in SAH

R. Higashida and D. Kuhne

Indications for endovascular treatment of patients who present with an intracranial aneurysm include (1) previous unsuccessful attempt at surgical clipping, (2) an aneurysm that is not surgically accessible, (3) medically high-risk patients, and (4) aneurysm's without a well defined neck.

The technique uses a transfemoral approach under general anesthesia with continuous neurological monitoring. The most widely used occlusion devices are detachable silicone or latex balloons, platinum coils (e.g. Guglielmi detachable coils, or GDCs). In patients with giant and/or fusiform aneurysms, a balloon test occlusion can first be done to ensure that the patient can tolerate occlusion of the major artery. In all cases a post-occlusion arteriogram should be done to document that the aneurysm has been excluded from the circulation.

Higashida and colleagues at the University of California San Francisco Medical Center are now treating 80% of all types of intracranial aneurysms (SAH and unruptured) by endovascular techniques. This group has treated 444 cerebral aneurysm cases which included 116 (26%) with giant aneurysms (>2.5 cm diameter), 253 (57%) who presented with mass effect, 145 (33%) with SAH, 24 (5%) with traumatic aneurysms, 15 (3%) with transient ischemic attacks (TIA), and 7 (2%) with rupture a of carotid cavernous aneurysm leading to fistula. Patients ranged in age from 3 months to 86 years. Three hundred twenty two patients had an aneurysm in the anterior circulation. One hundred twenty two had an aneurysm in the posterior circulation. Detachable balloons were used in 313 cases, microcoils in 13 cases, and GDC coils in 118 cases.

This endovascular approach was able to obliterate the aneurysm while preserving the parent artery in 51% of cases. Complications included stroke (7.9%), TIA (8.1%), hemorrhage (2.9%), and subtotal occlusion of less than 90% (12.6%). Mortality was 5.4%.

The risks and benefits of endovascular therapy are still best seen when individual patient cases are described. One case in this series was a 25-year-old female with severe retro-orbital pain, diplopia, 6th cranial nerve palsy, and a giant, ectatic cavernous aneurysm. The patient had a 3.5 cm diameter aneurysm with no well defined neck. This patient is an example of a fusiform aneurysm with no neck, therefore the balloon is chosen. The patient was systemically anticoagulated, and a balloon was placed into the cervical internal carotid artery from a transfemoral approach. The balloon was inflated for 30 minutes to have stasis of blood flow (Fig. 2). Neurological testing was done for 30 minutes to ensure that the patient had adequate collateral blood flow. Two detachable balloons were then placed across the base of the aneurysm and the cervical carotid artery for thrombosis of the aneurysm (Fig. 3). The 6-month follow-up CT scan showed thrombosis of the aneurysm and alleviation of the mass effect. The patient's symptoms resolved completely and she continues to do well at 10 years of follow-up with complete thrombosis and alleviation of her symptoms.

A very effective approach to treating patients with smaller aneurysms is with electrolytically detachable coils. In cases where the aneurysm has a well-defined

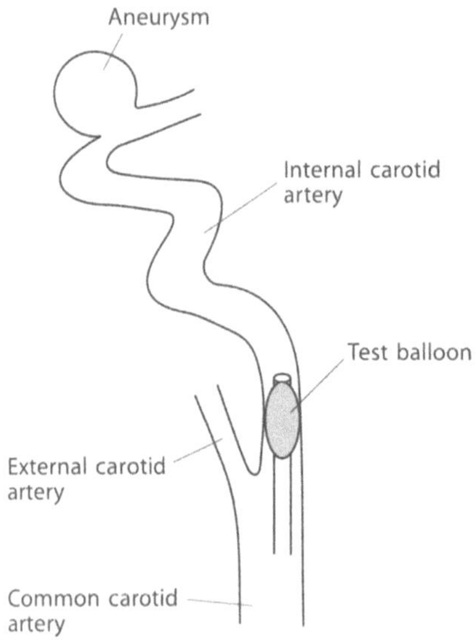

Fig. 2. Placement of test balloon for giant cavernous aneurysm

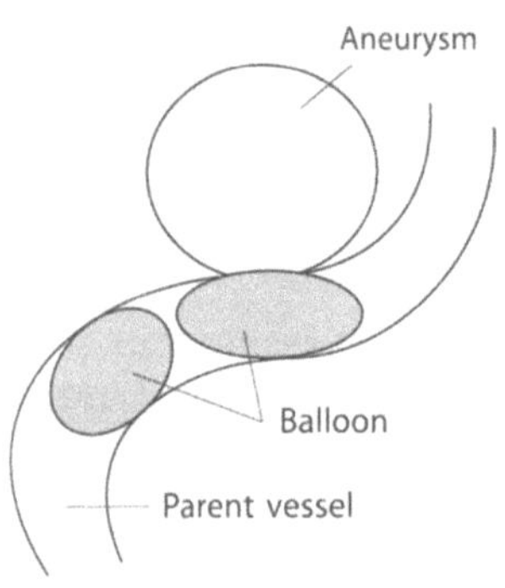

Fig. 3. Placement of balloons for thrombosis of giant cavernous aneurysm

neck, a microcatheter can be passed up from a transfemoral approach, with the tip of the catheter placed in the central lumen of the aneurysm. Platinum electrolytic coils are then advanced directly into the aneurysm for occlusion (Fig. 4). Once the coil is within the aneurysm, a small current is run through the coil juncture, the coil is detached by this current, and the guide wire is withdrawn. The positive current on the platinum coil promotes thrombosis of the aneurysmal lumen. The treatment goal is tight packing of the aneurysm and preservation of the parent artery (Fig. 5).

This approach was used in a 47-year-old woman with acute SAH and a 12 ¥ 16 mm internal carotid artery aneurysm, in grade II neurological condition. The frontal arteriogram showed that the aneurysm neck measured approximately 4 mm in diameter (Fig. 6). Neurosurgical exploration was undertaken but it

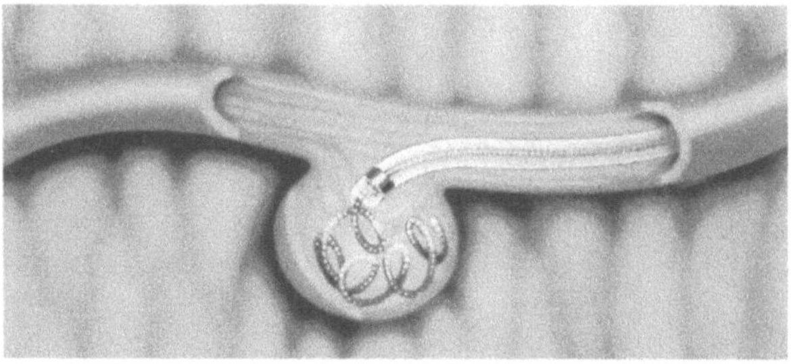

Fig. 4. Placement of microcatheter and electrolytic detachable coils

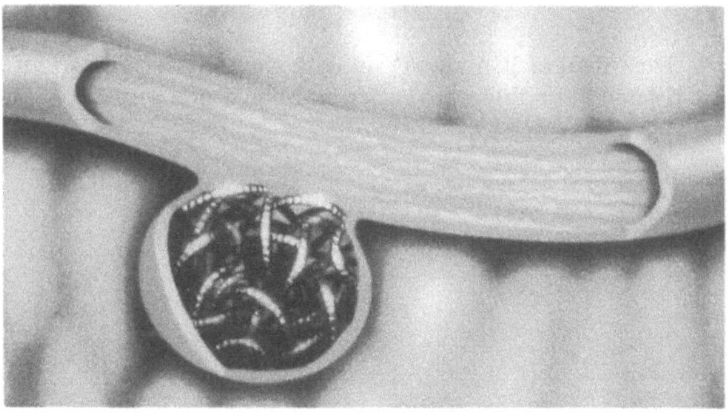

Fig. 5. Aneurysm lumen packed with electrolytic detachable coils

was not possible to clip the aneurysm because the neck extended into the cavernous sinus. The patient was referred for endovascular therapy. A microcatheter was placed through the internal carotid artery, and the tip of the microcatheter was navigated under fluoroscopy into the central lumen of the aneurysm. The lumen was filled with 6 electrolytically detachable coils, and the aneurysm was completely obliterated with preservation of the supraclinoid carotid artery and the intracranial blood flow (Fig. 6).

The youngest patient treated was a 3-month-old infant with massive hydrocephalus, and mass effect in the posterior fossa, and a large, partially thrombosed aneurysm which arose off the PICA artery (Fig. 7). The aneurysm could not be clipped and the patient was referred for endovascular therapy. A microcatheter was placed through the distal vertebral artery, navigated into the PICA artery, and placed into the aneurysm lumen. The aneurysm was filled with 6 GDC coils and successfully occluded.

A multi-institution GDC trial has been conducted [8]. Patients were eligible if they were not surgical candidates, had aneurysms in locations not surgically accessible, presented with anticipated surgical difficulty, had previous surgical failure, or refused surgery. This trial enrolled 735 patients ranging in age from 3 months to 90 years. Seventy percent were female, and 30% were male. The largest proportion of patients were referred for cavernous carotid (120) or basilar artery aneurysms (187). Forty-eight percent (356) of these patients had ruptured aneu-

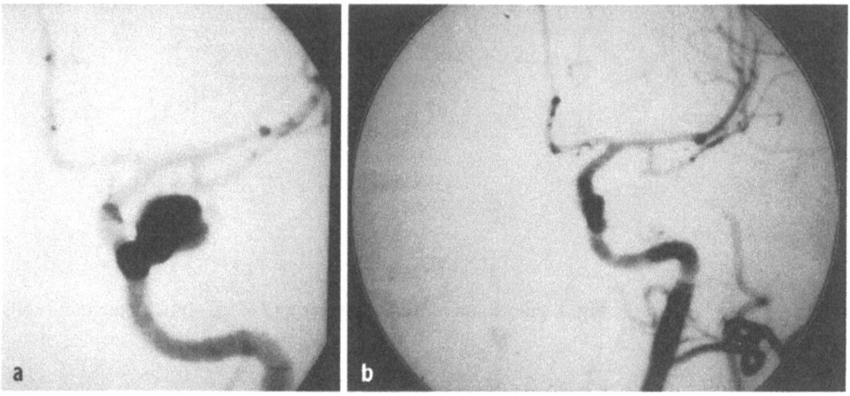

Fig. 6. Treatment of ICA aneurysm with electrolytic coils. **a** 12 × 16 mm aneurysm before treatment. **b** Aneurysm obliterated after placement of 6 coils

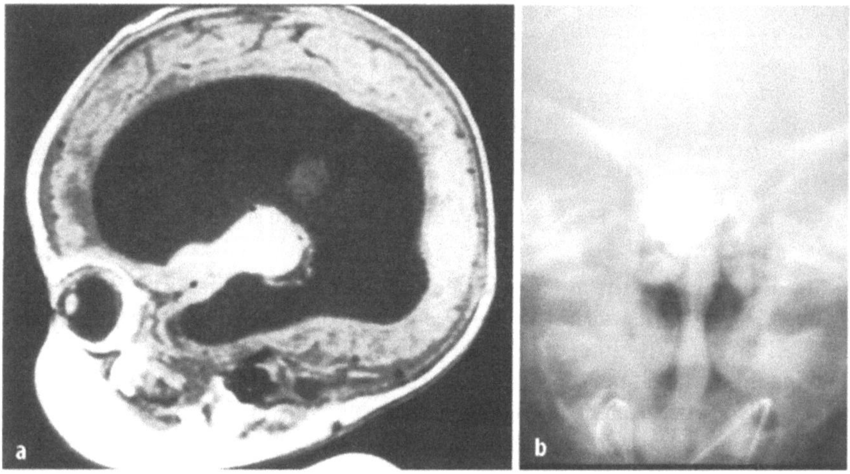

Fig. 7. GDC coil treatment of PICA aneurysm in an Infant. **a** Aneurysm before treatment. **b** Plain skull x-ray showing aneurysm packed with coils

rysms. Thirty-one percent of these ruptured aneurysms were acute and were treated within 15 days of bleeding. Seventeen percent were treated at later than 15 days. Aneurysms had not ruptured in 52% of patients (379). These included 53 giant (over 25 mm), 280 large (11–25 mm), and 46 asymptomatic aneurysms. Seventy-eight percent of patients were Hunt and Hess grade 1,2 or 3. Fifty-one percent of aneurysms treated were smaller than 10 mm, 38% were 11–25 mm, and 11% were greater than 25 mm. Only one procedure was performed in 80% of cases. Where more procedures were needed, the cause was either staged retreatment, recanalization, or regrowth of the aneurysm. A mean of 5.6 coils were placed per procedure (range 1–42).

Immediate occlusion can be achieved with a high degree of certainty, if the aneurysm measured less than 10 mm and the neck was less than 4 mm. The GDC technique in this group achieved a greater than 90% occlusion in 80% of cases. If the aneurysm measured 11 to 25 mm and the neck measured less than 4 mm, greater than 90% occlusion was achieved in 82% of cases. Occlusion was achieved in 86% of cases where the aneurysm was larger than 25 mm with a neck less than 4 mm. At 6 months follow-up, the GDC technique in this group achieved occlusion of over 90% of the lesion in 87% of patients with aneurysms smaller than 10 mm, 76% of patients with aneurysms 11–25 mm, and 78% of patients with aneurysms larger than 25 mm.

Mortality was 15.1% of patients with ruptured aneurysms. Of these, 10.8% were cerebrovascular deaths and 4.3% were due to other causes. Mortality for patients with unruptured aneurysms was 5.6%, with 4.0% due to cerebrovascular causes and 1.6% to other causes. Device-related adverse events totaled 8.7% (64 cases). Cerebral embolism related to the procedure accounted for most of these problems (34 or 4.6% of cases). There was a 1.2% incidence of intracranial bleeds, a 1% incidence of thrombosis, a 0.5% incidence of worsening symptoms, and a 0.5% incidence of aneurysm perforations. The periprocedural rebleed rates were 3.7% for ruptured aneurysms and 1.1% for unruptured aneurysms. Later rebleed rates at 6 months after treatment were 3.3% for ruptured aneurysms and 2.1% for unruptured aneurysms.

The advantages to GDC treatment for endovascular therapy are that it can be done under local anesthesia, and this technique thus allows for continuous neurological monitoring, that it is technically easier than balloon occlusion, that the coil may protect from early rebleeding, and that the coils are retrievable. Disadvantages are occasional subtotal occlusion (particularly for large and wide-neck aneurysms) and occasional coil compaction. There is also a risk of microemboli when coils are being placed into aneurysms that already have thrombus. There is also a small risk of the coil unraveling and going into the parent artery.

A major advantage to endovascular treatment is that it requires significantly less surgical time and shorter hospital stays. Recovery time is also significantly shorter (Table 2).

These endovascular methods are also becoming accepted in Europe because this approach allows the occlusion of aneurysms with minimal, if any, trauma to the brain and without the potential risk of craniotomy and surgical vessel preparation. Kuhne et al have used GDC coils to treat 179 patients with 202 aneurysms, including 147 small, 47 large, 6 giant, and 5 fusiform [9–11]. An addi-

Table 2. Intracranial aneurysm treatment

	Surgery	Interventional therapy
Hosoitalization time	6–10 days	3–4 days
Recovery time	6–8 weeks	1–2 weeks
Total cost	$ 45,000–60,000	$ 12,000–16,000

tional 15 asymptomatic aneurysms were treated surgically. Eighty four were in the anterior circulation, and 108 were in the posterior circulation. Of these patients, 179 had a history of hemorrhage, 23 were asymptomatic, and 34 were referred after failed surgical attempts. Treatment was 1 day to 3 weeks after bleeding.

Complete occlusion was achieved in 160 of 202 aneurysms. Thirty two aneurysms had neck remnants, 5 had only partial occlusions, and 5 had closure of the parent artery. Other complications included 9 cases of hemorrhage during treatment, 2 hemorrhages after treatment, 4 coil displacements, 16 thromboemboli, and 6 secondary occlusions of the parent artery. Complete recovery at 6–9 months after treatment occurred in 60/64 (94%) patients who were HH grade 1 at the time of treatment, 46/56 (82%) patients who were grade 2, 30/37 (81%) patients who were grade 3, 13/29 (45%) patients who were grade 4, and 6/16 (38%) patients who were grade 5. There also appeared to be a decreased frequency of recurrent hemorrhages in patients who were grade 4 or 5. Nine patients (5%) survived with permanent deficits, and 7 (3.9%) died.

Follow-up examinations were done after 12–18 months in 81 aneurysms. Four of 58 small and four of 17 medium sized aneurysms had minor refilling of the neck of the aneurysm. Five of six giant aneurysms had recanalized. The results were acceptable in terms of treatment, risks, and treatment-related mortality. Early GDC occlusion of grade 3 or 4 patients appears to reduce the risk of recurrent hemorrhage and associated complications. Coil obliteration of ruptured aneurysms also facilitates effective therapy against vasospasm.

Conclusion

Subarachnoid hemorrhage remains one of the most important problems in neurosurgery and neurology. Early surgical or endovascular treatment is recommended in most cases. Prospective data comparing surgery and interventional endovascular therapies for SAH do not exist. The current standard of care is emergent neurosurgical evaluation of the patient and early surgery. In the few centers where endovascular procedures are performed with high success rates and low morbidity/mortality, therapeutic options are usually assessed by the surgeon and interventional radiologist together. In some centers traditional surgical approaches are being replaced by less traumatic endovascular therapy in many cases. Indications for endovascular treatment of ruptured intracranial aneurysms include a location that is not surgically accessible, especially in posterior circulation; fusiform aneurysms, a patient in poor condition or advanced age, aneurysms associated with arteriovenous malformations, multiple bilateral aneurysms, partially clipped aneurysms or failed surgery, or severe vasospasm. One major advantage of surgery is that aneurysm rupture during treatment can be better controlled under surgical conditions but may be difficult to control with endovascular techniques. Careful evaluation of patients in a controlled manner will be needed to optimize the selection, timing, and combination of therapies.

References

1. Kassell NF, Torner JC, Jane JA, et al (1990) The International Cooperative Study on the Timing of Aneurysm Surgery. Part 2: Surgical results. J Neurosurgery 73(1):37–47
2. Ohman J, Heiskanen O (1989) Timing of operation for ruptured supratentorial aneurysms: a prospective randomized study. J Neurosurgery 70(1):55–60
3. Unpublished data from the data bank of 1993–1994 CVD study group, Nagoya University
4. Tsuji T, Cook DA, Weir BK, et al (1996) Effect of clot removal on cerebrovascular contraction after subarachnoid hemorrhage in the monkey: pharmacological study. Heart & Vessels 11(2):69–79
5. Findlay JM, Kassell NF, Weir BKA, et al (1995) A randomized trial of intraoperative, intracisternal tissue plasminogen activator for prevention of vasospasm. Neurosurgery 37: 168–178
6. Shitamichi M, Ogasawara T, Ara S, et al (1994) Attempt of the intra-operative head shaking method with t-PA for the treatment of vasospasm following aneurysmal SAH. Proceedings of 10th Spasm Symposium in Kyoto, 1994. Chugai Igakusha, Tokyo pp 284–288
7. Fujii Y, Takeuchi S, Sasaki O, et al (1996) Ultra-early rebleeding in spontaneous subarachnoid hemorrhage. J Neurosurg 84:35–42
8. Vinuela F, Duckwiler G, Mawad M (1997) Guglielmi detachable coil embolization of acute intracranial aneurysm: Perioperative anatomical and clinical outcome in 403 patients. J Neurosurg 86:475–482
9. Nahser HC, Kuhne D (1994) Experience with Guglielmi detachable coils in the treatment of intracranial aneurysms. Zentralblatt für Neurochirurgie Suppl:34
10. Kuhne D, Nahser HC, Henkes H (1995) Treatment of intracranial aneurysms with Guglielmi detachable coils. Neuroradiology Suppl 37:423–424
11. Nahser HC, Kuhne D, Henkes H, et al (1996) Treatment of intracranial aneurysms after subarachnoid hemorrhage with Guglielmi detachable coils. Neurology 46(2):370 (Abst)

Vasospasm Following Subarachnoid Hemorrhage: Medical and Transvascular Treatment

D. Wecht, J. Eskridge, M. Findlay, and J. Torner

Introduction

Vasospasm is a common sequela of aneurysmal subarachnoid hemorrhage (SAH). Early surgery and cisternal irrigation facilitate care of the patient in vasospasm, but meticulous attention to the details and timing of interventions is critical, and care must be highly individualized. The incidence of aneurysmal SAH is 6–16 per 100,000 population, and angiographic vasospasm is seen in about 75% of such patients, generally between days 4 and 10 following SAH [1–4]. Symptomatic vasospasm is seen in about 30% of cases [5].

One of the most important risk factors associated with vasospasm is the thickness and distribution of the clot. Current medical and endovascular approaches attempt to reduce or prevent vasospasm by reducing the presence of clot. More direct transvascular approaches with balloon angioplasty are appropriate when medical management fails, and topical application of thrombolytics may have a role in some cases. Major questions about SAH treatment remain, however, and carefully designed clinical trials will be needed to answer them.

Medical Treatment of Vasospasm After SAH

Vasospasm is delayed cerebral arterial (and arteriolar) constriction following SAH. It is commonly seen following aneurysmal SAH but also can occur in other conditions. The main risk factors for vasospasm are related to the thickness and distribution of extravasated (subarachnoid) blood in the basal cisterns. The most notable predictor of vasospasm risk is the thickness and distribution of clot noted on computed tomographic (CT) scan.

Fisher et al. showed that patients with thick basal clot on CT have a higher incidence of angiographic and clinical vasospasm than those with no obvious hemorrhage or with mild hemorrhage on CT [6] (Table 1). Interestingly, Grade IV patients with intraparenchymal or intraventricular clot did not have a very high incidence of either angiographic or clinical vasospasm.

Angiographic vasospasm peaks at days 6–8 after SAH. Clinical vasospasm appears 3–4 days after SAH, and peaks at 7–9 days, and ebbs by 10–12 days. Clinical changes may include headache, altered level of consciousness, focal neurologic deficits, and seizures. The course of clinical vasospasm can last for up to three weeks. This suggests that a spasmogen related to extravasated blood is the real

Table 1. Relationship between subarachnoid hemorrhage and vasospasm

CT grade	CT evidence of SAH	No. of cases	Vasospasm incidence	
			Angiographic	Clinical
	None	11	2	0
I	Diffuse mild hemorrhage	7	0	0
II	Localized clots or thick layers of blood in cisterns or fissures (1 mm or greater)	24	23	23

Adapted from Fisher, 1980

culprit. Attempts to identify the spasmogen(s) responsible for post-SAH vasospasm have produced several candidates. Oxyhemoglobin is one possibility. Other contributing factors may include loss of autoregulation, maximal dilatation of parenchymal vessels distally, decreased regional cerebral blood flow, or impaired microcirculation.

Histologically, acute vasospasm is accompanied by a number of characteristic changes. These include reduced ratio of lumen-to-wall thickness; loss of the characteristic flat shape of the endothelial cells; corrugation of the intima in the direction of flow, and smooth muscle contraction. If vasospasm becomes chronic, there are typically inflammatory changes, subendothelial proliferation, and myonecrosis.

Medical Management

Patients who have suffered an aneurysmal SAH should be admitted to the neurological intensive care unit for close neurological observation. Noninvasive monitoring should include pulse oximetry and electrocardiogram. Invasive monitoring typical includes an arterial linc, Foley catheter, central venous line or Swan-Ganz catheter to monitor pulmonary capillary wedge pressure, and intracranial pressure monitoring for patients who are below GCS 9, preferably with ventriculostomy. Diagnostic adjuncts may include transcranial doppler to correlate with clinical impression and CT scan if there is suspicion of an infarct or hemorrhage.

Patients suitable for surgery should have early surgery. Aneurysm clipping is still the gold standard and facilitates treatment of any post-SAH vasospasm. It should be emphasized that early surgery is not associated with an increased risk for spasm. Surgery also allows for irrigation of basal cisterns and instillation of papaverine or thrombolytics.

The therapeutic approach varies depending on the patient's clinical condition. Treatment goals are to improve blood flow and oxygen delivery by improving perfusion pressure and decreasing blood viscosity. Patients who are at risk for vasospasm but not yet symptomatic should be hydrated vigorously and treated with calcium channel blockers such as nimodipine, unless they are hypotensive.

Avoid arterial hypotension and hold antihypertensive therapies. Patients should be monitored by clinical examination and TCD.

Patients who are clearly symptomatic should be treated more aggressively with hyperdynamic therapy. Hypervolemic hypertensive hemodilution (HHH) therapy includes administration of crystalloids or colloids (5% albumin), to a pulmonary wedge pressure of 12–16 mmHg and systolic blood pressure of 160–200 mmHg. Dopamine is used to increase cardiac output and cerebral perfusion pressure. Hematocrit is kept at 30–35, which can usually be accomplished by ample hydration without the need for phlebotomy. Patients who are not following commands, generally with GCS below 9, should receive an ICP monitor, preferably with a ventriculostomy to permit cerebrospinal fluid drainage. Avoid sustained hyperventilation.

Endovascular intervention should be considered for patients who are clearly progressing despite maximal medical intervention. Endovascular treatment is best if attempted within 12–18 hours of a new deficit. Papaverine can produce initially good results, but the effect tends to be transient [7–9]. Angioplasty may be more appropriate if the patient has well-identified lesions that are accessible with minimal morbidity.

Complications of aggressive treatment of post-SAH vasospasm can include brain edema from over perfusion, progressive infarction, seizure, or hemorrhage. Non-neurologic complications can include pulmonary edema, electrolyte disturbances, or infection.

Future directions in care of these patients include ongoing work with intracisternal thrombolytics, brain protective agents such as free radical scavengers, endovascular treatment, estrogen therapy in postmenopausal women, and intrathecal papaverine.

Transvascular Treatment of Vasospasm Following SAH

When endovascular management of vasospasm following SAH is indicated, there is widespread agreement that both technique and timing are crucial. Balloon angioplasty should be used to gradually dilate the area of spasm. Use multiple inflations and deflations, in at least 4 or 5 steps (Fig. 1). Results are generally better with this approach than with attempting to go to full inflation immediately. Stepwise angioplasty can provide excellent relief of severe vasospasm (Fig. 2).

Acute spasm is easier to dilate than chronic spasm, so earlier angioplasty is also safer. Once vasospasm is clearly developing, as indicated by TCD, optimal medical therapy should include hypervolemic hypertensive hemodilution (HHH). If this is not sufficient, perform angioplasty before the area of spasm is too fibrotic to open.

Angioplasty should be done using a transfemoral approach and full heparinization. General anesthesia is recommended. Digital road-mapping is essential.

Only dilate proximally. The target area for dilation is typically the supraclinoid internal carotid artery, the proximal middle cerebral artery (MCA) and the verte-

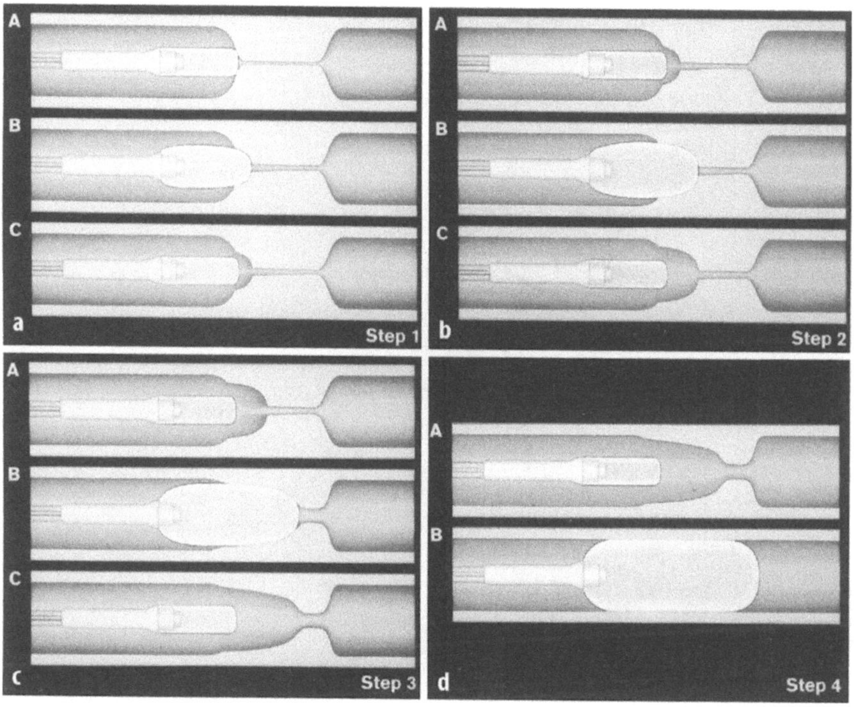

Fig. 1a–d. Stepwise balloon angioplasty of vasospasm

bro basilar artery. Distal areas can be treated with papaverine. Do not dilate beyond the M2, A1, and P1 segments.

A key safety rule is not to use a balloon larger than the artery. As dilation progresses distally, smaller balloons should be used, to 3–4mm diameter. Dilatation of vessels smaller than this diameter is not recommended. The lowest possible pressure should be used for dilation.

Difficult areas are typically the supraclinoid carotid and the distal veretebral arteries. Unfortunately, these are also the first areas that must be opened. Opening only one vertebral artery is usually sufficient.

Difficult to reach areas can be approached by putting a wire in the balloon to curve the balloon up and into the segment (Fig. 3). The newly available stealth catheter from Target Therapeutics is a 3 mm balloon with a 10 mm length and can be used for more difficult areas (Fig. 4).

Intra-arterial papaverine has limited usefulness. The effect lasts only about 24 hours, and rapid infusion raises the blood pressure and the ICP [10]. Papaverine (infused at 300 mg per vessel in 120 cc at 3 cc/min) can be used in conjunction with angioplasty for more long-term protection.

There is some controversy regarding the appropriate use of balloon angioplasty to relieve post-SAH vasospasm in comatose patients. Coma is due to damage to the ascending reticular activating system and to both hemispheres, so both ar-

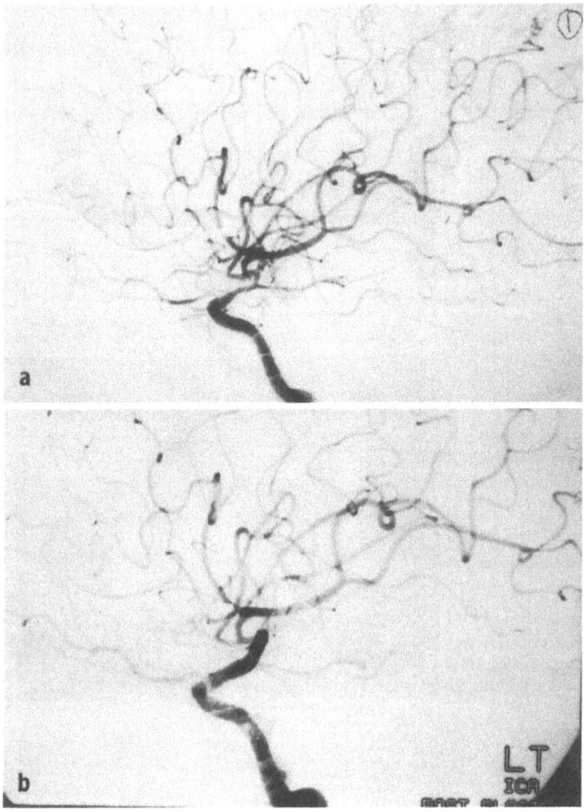

Fig. 2a, b. Vasospasm before and after balloon angioplasty

eas must be treated. The brain coma center is supplied by thalamoperforators coming off the P1 arteries. In 85% of people these anastamose [11], so the therapeutic goal is to open at least one P1 segment. In the comatose patient, a reasonable approach is to dilate the vertebrobasilar system, at least one P1, and the anterior circulation spasm.

Angioplasty can produce significant improvement in comatose patients. In a recent series, angioplasty was done within 18 hours of symptom onset in 41 of 50 patients. Thirty three (66%) improved at least 2 levels in coma scale or motor strength in 48 hours. Complications included three procedure deaths, one branch occlusion, two patients who rebled because their aneurysms were not clipped or protected in any way. Five patients were Grade V [12]. A similar series of 120 patients treated with angioplasty plus papaverine showed improvement in 70 (58%) [13]. Long-term follow-up angiograms in three patients who had received vertebrobasilar system angioplasties showed that arteries were still open after 18 months. Clinically, there has been no neurological deterioration in 80 patients treated more than one year ago. Twenty patients treated more than three years ago remain normal on TCD.

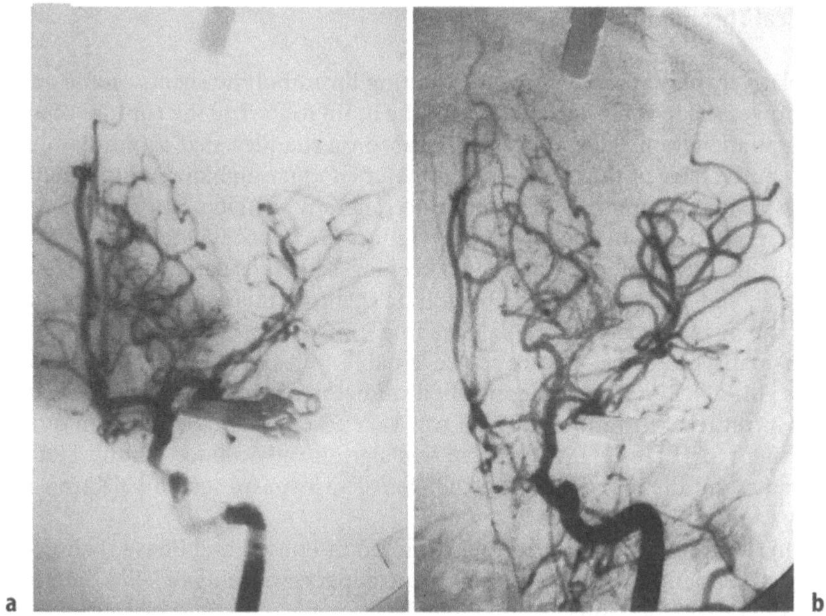

Fig. 3a, b. Wire-guided balloon angioplasty

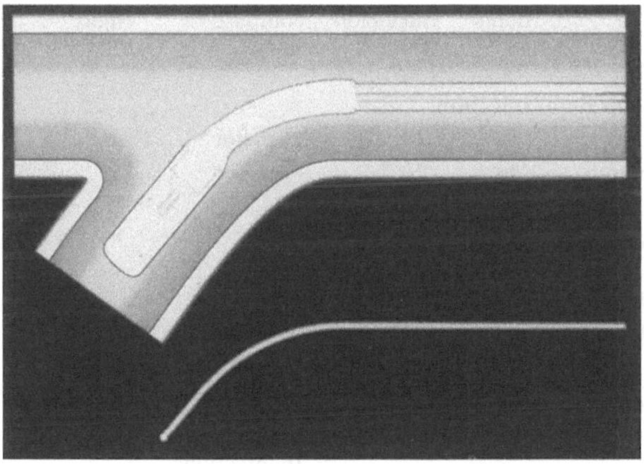

Fig. 4. New "Stealth" catheter

Topical Thrombolytics

A relatively new approach involves putting thrombolytic agents on the outside of blood vessels in the brain and within the brain following the rupture of an intracranial aneurysm. This approach is based on the idea that rapid dissolution of clots at the base of the brain around major conducting blood vessels may reduce vasospasm. Eliminating clots more peripherally distributed over the convexity and between the hemispheres may reduce SAH encephalopathy. Lysing clots within the ventricular system and keeping catheters patent may facilitate ICP control. The danger of giving fibrinolytic agents in this way following a major hemorrhagic injury is intracranial bleeding.

In many cases, vasospasm is preventable by early removal of subarachnoid clots [14–17]. Randomized, controlled studies in a primate model of SAH showed that intrathecal thrombolytic TPA was very effective at clearing even quite large confluent SAH [18–21]. Vasospasm was significantly reduced in the TPA-treated animals, and the morphological changes of vasospasm seen on electron microscopy were similarly reduced.

This approach has been further explored in Phase I and Phase II clinical trials [22–24]. Patients were given a single intraoperative bolus of TPA, then multiple postoperative injections via a catheter left in subarachnoid space at time of aneu-

Table 2. Effect of topical TPA on rate of severe vasospasm in 400 patients with severe SAH (Findlay)

Non-randomized or uncontrolled trials of thrombolysis for VSP prevention (1991 – present)							
First author	# Patients	# Patients thick clots	Treatment complications	All angio. VSP	Angio. severe VSP	Symp. VSP	Infarcts due to VSP
Intraop. Bolus injection							
Findlay	15	18	1 major	8	1	1	1
Ohman	30	20	2 major	16	0	10	10
Stolke	20	20	0	?	?	1	1
Seifert	52	52	0	?	?	4 (8%)	?
Postop. Cisternal injections or infusions							
Kodama	106	106	3 (3%)	?	?	3 (3%)	?
Zabrarnski	10	10	1 minor	9	1	0	?
Mizoi	30	30	3 minor	4	1 (3%)	0	0
Usui	82	74	1 bleeding/ 16 infections	?	?	13 (16%)	7 (9%)
Sasaki	46	31	4 (7%)	40 (87%)	0	12 (16%) 1 severe	4 (9%)
Postendovascular ablation intrathecal injections							
Kinugasa	12	9	–	2	0	0	0
Totals	403	365	31 (8%)	55%	2%	11%	10%

rysm repair. There was continuous irrigation through the ventricular system into the subarachnoid space before drainage. Intrathecal/intraventricular injections following aneurysm ablation with solid polymer. (This approach would be inappropriate to use with GDC coil repair, which depends on thrombosis of the broken aneurysm).

Overall, 400 patients have been treated. Most had thick, severe hemorrhages and were at high risk for severe vasospasm. About half of patients had vasospasm despite treatment, but severe vasospasm was extremely uncommon, and the incidence of symptomatic and vasospastic infarction was far lower than expected using historical cohort controls (Table 2).

This work was continued in a double-blind, randomized, placebo-controlled trial of 100 patients with aneurysms and severe intracranial hemorrhage. The major endpoint was severe angiographic vasospasm.

The results showed a reduction in vasospasm incidence in treated patients, but this reached statistical significance only in the subgroup with thick clots. There were trends toward reduced TCD velocities and reduced requirement for HHH therapy. There was no significant difference in outcomes, but there were trends toward more good recovery and fewer deaths in treated patients. There was no difference in the complication rate due to bleeding [25] (Table 1). Thus, it appears that this method facilitates the management of large intraventricular hemorrhage. It is not possible to determine if it improves outcome.

Open Questions About Vasospasm and Subarachnoid Hemorrhage

SAH incidence has remained constant while other forms of stroke have declined in incidence. Prevention of SAH has yet to be proven. Strategies that may have benefit include screening of high-risk populations such as those with a positive family history by angiography, helical CT or magnetic resonance angiography, controlling hypertension, smoking cessation, and obliteration by surgical or endovascular procedures of unruptured aneurysms. Only hypertension control has been shown to decrease risk of stroke [26]. However, none of the trials had specific endpoints of SAH.

Once a SAH occurs there are many prognostic factors that influence outcome. not only the initial hemorrhage can cause death and disability, but also recurrent hemorrhage, vasospasm-related ischemia and medical complications can occur. Factors such as neurological grade, amount of SAH blood on CT, and physiologic measures such as glucose level predict outcome [27].

Attempts to prevent rebleeding have demonstrated that bedrest and antihypertensive therapy of reducing blood pressure after the SAH are not effective [28]. Carotid ligation reduced recurrent hemorrhage but was applicable only to a limited number of patients [28]. Antifibrinolytic agents decreased rebleeding but increased the risk of cerebral ischemia by preserving the spasmogenic properties of the blood [29]. Early aneurysmal surgical clipping in the first 3 days prevented rebleeding. The use of early increased from about 20% in the early 1980's to 75% in recent studies [30].

In the treatment of vasospasm and its associated ischemia there are two regimens utilized predominantly. One is use of calcium channel blocking agents such as nimodipine. Benefits of calcium channel blocking agents have been demonstrated in randomized clinical trials [31]. Another therapy used is hypervolemia-hemodilution-hypertension (HHH). These therapies are utilized once the aneurysm has been clipped and are intended to counteract the reduction in cerebral blood flow from vasospasm. HHH has been studies only in observational studies, but use of HHH either as prophylaxis or as therapy has increased to about 80% in recent studies [32, 33]. Angioplasty has also been used as a rescue therapy, and reported efficacy is also based on observational studies.

Currently for patients who suffer a SAH, 55% have a good recovery, 25% are disabled, and 20% die. While the initial hemorrhage is still the primary cause of death and disability, vasospasm and medical complications remain as challenges. There has been a steady decline in mortality and disability in the clinical trials reported.

However, in the United States, the trend in mortality showed a decline from 1970 to 1985 with little improvement since then (Fig. 5) [34]. The community survival rate is much lower than the hospital and clinical trial rates. There needs to be more education of the population and of primary care physicians on the importance of early recognition, prompt diagnosis, and rapid referral. Also, preventive strategies such as high-risk screening should be considered. Epidemiologic studies of smoking, hypertension, alcohol use, oral contraceptives, family history, and aneurysm size and location need to be done. The international Study of Unruptured Intracranial Aneurysms is underway. it will include over 5,000 patients and seeks to identify factors related to SAH. Surgical and endovascular treatment of unruptured aneurysms also needs evaluation in a multi-center clinical trial. A prospective study evaluating blood pressure control and smoking cessation might also be warranted.

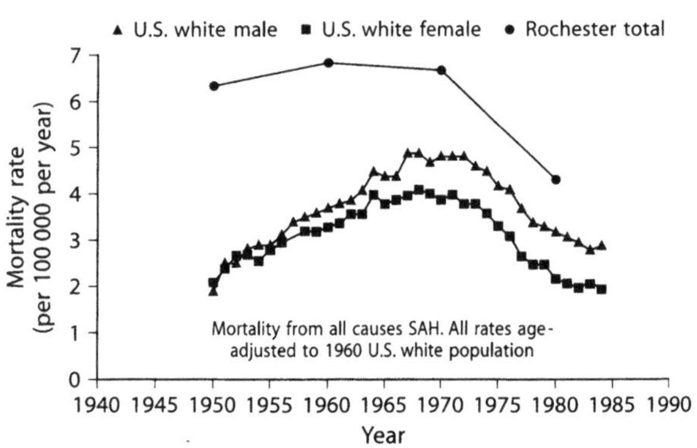

Fig. 5. U.S. Mortality from SAH, 1940–1990

Conclusion

Unanswered questions in the prevention and treatment of aneurysmal SAH include:

1) Identification of high risk populations for aneurysms
2) Usefulness of helical CT and MRI for diagnosis and prevalence
3) Identification of genetic, hormonal, and behavioral factors that lead to rupture
4) Effect of modification of risk factors on SAH incidence
5) Evaluation of medical and surgical procedures for unruptured aneurysms
6) Recognition of SAH and improvement of referral
7) Evaluation of therapies for SAH such as endovascular treatment, vasospasm prophylaxis and treatment, neuroprotection during surgery and vasospasm, and best medical, intensive care management of complications.

The challenges are in identifying those high-risk persons who will have a rupture and who will have a poor prognosis. Studies may need to use mechanistic endpoints such as helical CT to monitor size and shape of aneurysmal change and TCD or angiography to measure vessel diameter in vasospasm. Well-designed studies with adequate sample size, uniform protocols, standardized treatments, and complete ascertainment of standardized endpoints are needed to determine the best prevention and treatment of SAH.

References

1. Kassell NF, Torner JC, Haley EC, et al (1990) The International Cooperative Study on the Timing of Aneurysm Surgery. Part 1: Overall management results. J Neurosurgery 73: 18–36
2. Drake CG (1981) Progress in cerebrovascular disease. Management of cerebral aneurysm. Stroke 12: 273–283
3. Phillips LH 2d, Whisnant JP, O'Fallon WM, et al (1980) The unchanging pattern of subarachnoid hemorrhage in a community. Neurology 30: 1034–1040
4. Weir B (ed) (1987) Aneurysms Affecting the Nervous System, Baltimore, Williams and Wilkins
5. Mayberg M (1996) Intracranial arterial spasm. In: Neurosurgery (2nd edition), New York, McGraw-Hill, pp 2245–2254
6. Fisher CM, Kistler JP, Davis JM (1980) Relation of cerebral vasospasm to subarachnoid hemorrhage visualized by computerized tomographic scanning. Neurosurgery 6(1): 1–9
7. Kassell NF, Helm G, Simmons N, et al (1992) Treatment of cerebral vasospasm with intra-arterial papaverine. J Neurosurgery 77: 848–852
8. Clouston JE, Numaguchi Y, Zoarski GH, et al (1995) Intraarterial papaverine infusion for cerebral vasospasm after subarachnoid hemorrhage. AJNR: Am J Neuroradiol 16: 27–38
9. Dion JE, Mathis JM, Vinuela F (1996) Endovascular Treatment of Cervicocerebral Aneurysms. In: Wilkins and Rengachary (eds) Neurosurgery, 2nd ed. McGraw-Hill Inc., New York, pp 2383–2403
10. McAuliffe W, Tounsend M, Eskridge JM, et al (1995) Intracranial pressure changes during papavrine infusion for vasospasm. J Neurosurg 83: 426–429
11. Eskridge JM, Newell DW, Winn HR (1994) Endovascular treatment of vasospasm. In: Advances in Neuroembolization Neurosurgery Clinics North America, WB Saunders, Philadelphia, PA, pp 437–448

12. Eskridge JM, McAuliffe W, Song J, et al. Treatment of vasospasm: results of first 50 patients. Neurosurgery (in press)
13. Eskridge JM (unpublished data)
14. Findlay JM, Weir BK, Steinke D, et al (1988) Effect of intrathecal thrombolytic therapy on subarachnoid clot and chronic vasospasm in a primate model of SAH. J Neurosurg 69: 723–735
15. Findlay JM, Weir BK, Gordon P, et al (1989) Safety and efficacy of intrathecal thrombolytic in a primate model of cerebral vasospasm. Neurosurg 24:4:491–498
16. Findlay JM, Weir BK, Kassell NF, et al (1991) Intracisternal recombinant tissue plasminogen activator after aneurysmal subarachnoid hemorrhage. J Neurosurg 75:181–188
17. Kinugasa K, Kamata I, Hirotsune N, et al (1995) Early treatment of subarachnoid hemorrhage after preventing rerupture of an aneurysm. J Neurosurg 83:34–41
18. Ohman J, Servo A, Heisdanen O (1991) Effect of intrathecal fibrinolytic therapy on clot lysis and vasospasm in patients with aneurysmal subarachnoid hemorrhage. J Neurosurg 75: 197–201
19. Stolke D, Seifert V (1992) Single intracisternal bolus of recombinant tissue plasminogen activator in patients with aneurysmal subarachnoid hemorrhage: preliminary assessment of efficacy and safety in an open clinical study. 30:6:877–881
20. Sasali T, Ohta T, Kikuchi H, et al (1994) A Phase II clinical trial of recombinant human tissue-type plasminogen activaator against cerebaral vasospasm after aneurysmal subarachnoid hemorrhage. Neurosurgery 35:4:597–605
21. Seifert V, Zimmermann M, Feldges A (1994) Prevention of delayed ischaemic deficits after aneurysmal subarachnoid haemorrhage by intrathecal bolus injection of tissue plasminogen activator (rTPA). Acta Neurochir 128:137–143
22. Sano K, Takakura K, Kassell N, et al (1990) Proceeding of the IVth Internatonal Conference on Cerebral Vasospasm (Chapter 10). In: Cerebral Vasospasm, University Of Tokyo Press, Tokyo, pp 292–296
23. Zabramski J, Spetzler R, Lee KS, et al (1991) Phase I trial of plasminogen activator for the prevention of vasospasm in patients with aneurysmal subarachnoid hemorrhage. J Neurosurg 75:189–196
24. Mizoi K, Yoshimoto T, Takahashi A et al (1993) Prospective study on the prevention of cerebral vasospasm by intrathecal fibrinolytic therapy with tissue-type plasminogen activator. J Neurosurg 78:430–437
25. Usui M, Saito N, Hoya K, et al (1994) Vasospasm prevention with postoperative intrathecal thrombolytic therapy: a retrospective comparison of urokinase, tissue plasminogen activator, and cisternal drainage alone. Neurosurgery 34:2:235–245
26. Collins R, Peto R, MacMahon S, et al (1990) Blood pressure, stroke, and coronary heart disease Part 2. Short-term reductions in blood pressures: overview of randomized drug trials in their epidemiologic context. Lancet 335:827–838
27. Lanzino G, Kassell N, Germanson T, et al (1993) Plasma glucose levels and outcome after subarachnoid hemorrhage. J Neurosurg 79:885–891
28. Sahs AL, Nibbelink DW, Torner JC, et al (eds) (1981) Aneurysmal Subarachnoid Hemorrhage. Report of the Cooperative Study. Baltimore, Urban and Schwarzenberg
29. Kassell NF, Haley EC, Torner JC (1986) Antifibrinolytic therapy in the treatment of aneurysmal subarachnoid hemorrhage. Current Neurosurgery 33:137–145
30. Kassell NF, Torner JC, Haley EC, Jane JA, et al (1990) The international cooperative study on the timing of aneurysm surgery. II. Surgical results. J Neurosurgery 73:37–47
31. Barker F, Ogilvy C (1996) Efficacy of prophylactic nimodipine for delayed ischemic deficit after subarachnoid hemorrhage: a meta-analysis. J Neurosurg 84:405–414
32. Haley E, Kassell N, Torner J (1993) A randomized controlled trial of high-dose intravenous nicardipine in aneurysmal subarachnoid hemorrhage. A report of the Cooperative Aneurysm Study. J Neurosurg 78:537–547
33. Kassell N, Haley E, Aperson-Hansen C, et al (1996) Randomized double-blind, vehicle-controlled trial of tirilazad mesylate in patients with aneurysmal subarachnoid hemorrhage: a comparative study in Europe, Australasia, and New Zealand. J Neurosurg 84:221–228
34. Ingall T, Whisnant J, Wiebers D, et al (1989) Has there been a decline in subarachnoid hemorrhage mortality? Stroke 20:718–724

Cytoprotective Drugs After Subarachnoid Hemorrhage

T. P. Bleck

Introduction

Many mechanisms have been postulated to account for vasospasm following subarachnoid hemorrhage (SAH). These include nitric oxide, oxygen-derived free radicals, endothelins, protein kinase C activation, changes in endothelial Ca^{2+} and K^{+} fluxes, increases in platelet-activating factor, and loss of smooth muscle phosphatases. Many of these different pathologic systems can be tied together. The excitatory amino acid systems can result in generation of free radicals. The systems that produce reperfusion injury can develop free radicals. Nitric oxide itself can function as a free radical and can increase the production of others. Lipid peroxidation can result in more extracellular glutamate release.

This complexity indicates that cytoprotection cannot be based simply on eliminating free radical production. Interfering with only one of these mechanisms would be unlikely to stop the entire process of neuronal necrosis.

Pathologic Mechanisms in Post-SAH Vasospasm

Free radicals themselves have a number of adverse effects. Lipid peroxidation has received the most research attention [1–5]. Excess extracellular free radicals also interfere with the removal of glutamate from the extracellular space, which can directly modulate N-methyl-D-aspartate (NMDA) receptor function. This would result in more calcium entry through the NMDA receptors. Voltage-sensitive calcium channels also may play a role in neuronal destruction.

Lipid peroxidation is an autocatalyzing reaction. The introduction of free radicals into the lipid membrane results in the production of portions of the membrane which are themselves free radicals. This reaction can then spread across the membrane and result in a new hole in the cell. While this is very useful as a defense against bacteria, it is deleterious to the maintenance neuronal integrity.

Cytoprotection is often considered a measure to be instituted after the onset of vasospasm, but its effective use requires prophylactic treatment before vasospasm has started. In many cases, beginning treatment after the vasospasm-associated injury has occurred is too late. The ideal is to have the patient's brain saturated with the cytoprotective substance before vasospasm begins, therefore preventing or diminishing the neuronal effects of delayed ischemia.

Standard Approaches to Cytoprotection

The standard cytoprotective treatments are calcium antagonists such as nimodipine [3] and nicardipine [6, 7] or free radical scavengers such as tirilizad [8]. The calcium antagonists are effective only at the voltage-sensitive calcium channels. They do not effect calcium entry through the NMDA receptor.

Nimodipine had been thought to protect against neuronal damage by antagonizing calcium-mediated vasospasm, but this appears not to be the case. Nimodipine treatment has no effect on vasospastic arterial caliber measured angiographically [9]. A recent metaanalysis confirms that there is a neuroprotective effect of nimodipine which appears to be neuroprotection in areas supplied by vasospastic arteries [10]. Nicardipine, in contrast, does appear to have a direct arterial relaxant effect [11]. A neuroprotective effect has been difficult to document but is thought to exist, because patients who receive nicardipine had less need for conventional hypertensive hemodilution therapy [12]. With regard to side effects, both of these drugs can produce hypotension. Nicardipine at the higher doses has also been associated with the high-output form of congestive heart failure, which can cause pulmonary edema [12].

New Pharmacologic Approaches

Pharmacologic approaches to reducing the damage caused by free radicals have included tirilazad mesylate, polyethylene glycol-conjugated superoxide dismutase (PEG-SOD), mannitol, carnitine, allopurinol, and prostaglandin manipulations [13–17]. Several of these substances are potentially useful but do not readily cross into the central nervous system (CNS) in sufficient concentrations to be useful.

Tirilazad has shown efficacy in several studies [18, 19]. It is an aminosteroid free radical scavenger, one of a group of compounds developed to duplicate the free-radical scavenging effect of methylprednisolone but without a glucocorticoid effect. This was accomplished by removing a hydroxyl group such that the molecule no longer fits the glucocorticoid receptor and therefore does not cause the usual steroid side effects.

The European/Australian and American tirilazad studies produced somewhat different results, which were apparently due to previously unappreciated aspects of tirilazad metabolism. These include: (1) women metabolize tirilazad much more rapidly than men, and (2) anticonvulsants induce tirilazad metabolism. The European/Australian SAH reported markedly beneficial effects of tirilazad, but most of the benefit was in men who were not receiving anticonvulsants [18]. A smaller positive effect was reported in the American trial [19]. In that study, the positive effect was statistically significant for men. A major difference between these two studies is that only about 40% of patients in the European/Australian trial were receiving phenytoin, but 80% of patients in the American trial were.

The European/Australian trial was a randomized, double-blind, vehicle-controlled study with tirilazad doses of 0.5, 2.0, or 6.0 mg/kg/day IV; 255 patients were randomized to each group and treated within 48 hours of SAH. This is an inadequate dose, and was based on animal studies suggesting that there was a U-shaped dose-response curve and that the best outcome in baboons was at 2.0 mg/kg/day. (We now appreciate that there seem to be wide differences in tirilazad metabolism among different species.) Subsequent clinical trials have used 10 and 15 mg/kg/day doses.

Patients in these trials were adults who had SAH associated with typical saccular aneurysms. Patients who were at risk because of other diseases or who were receiving other investigation drugs that might interfere with our ability to determine mechanism of action were excluded. In the European/Australian trial intravenous nimodipine was required unless it had to be stopped due to hypotension. In the American trial oral nimodipine was used. Other concurrent therapy could include HHT therapy and angioplasty but no steroids.

Overall outcome data (Table 1) showed that tirilazad produced a 43% reduction in death and a 21% increase in the percentage of patients with good outcomes after 3 months (Table 2). There was a trend toward better outcome in tirilazad patients presenting in all Hunt and Hess grades, although some of these groups were too small to reach statistical significance (Table 2). The greatest reduction in mortality was in patients who present as grade V (25% vs. 53%, P=0.02). Only the 6.0 mg dose affected mortality (Table 1).

Most of the positive effect occurred in male patients in the study, who had a 51% increase in good outcomes and an 89% decrease in mortality with 6.0 mg/kg/day tirilazad. Female patients had a 7% increase in good outcomes (P=0.06) and a 3% decrease in mortality (P=0.88). This difference is at least

Table 1. Overall outcome with tirilazad (6.0 mg/kg/day IV): Glasgow Outcome Score

	Tirilazad	Vehicle	Change	*P*
Dead	12%	21%	43%	0.01
Disabled	24%	26%	11%	0.64
Good	54%	53%	71%	0.02
Able to resume previous work	64%	52%	23%	0.01

Table 2. Percentage of patients with overall good outcomes (GDS = 1 at 3-month follow-up)

Presenting grade	Tirilazad (6.0 mg/kg/day)	Vehicle	*P*
I	82%	79%	0.67
II	70%	59%	0.15
III	37%	25%	0.43
IV	33%	22%	0.39
V	31%	15%	0.11

partly explained by the observation that tirilazad is metabolized more slowly in men and thus achieves higher therapeutic levels. Unfortunately, blood levels were not measured during most of this study, but data from studies of tirilazad in head injury support this possibility. Interestingly, the 6.0 mg dose was also associated with the fewest serious medical events related to the CNS (15% vs. 27% for vehicle, 20% for 0.6 mg and 26% for 2.0 mg). There did not appear to be any neurotoxicity associated with tirilazad. There had been concern among investigators that patients complaining of pain on injection or who develop phlebitis might be getting the drug, which would disrupt study blinding, but the data show that both the vehicle and vehicle plus drug can cause phlebitis.

The beneficial effect of tirilazad at 6.0 mg/kg/day was also apparent in a reduced need for therapeutic hypertension and hemodilution (9% vs. 15%, $P=0.018$). The question of optimal tirilazad dosing remains unsettled, but some useful insights can be gleaned from studies in head injury patients. This work suggested that outcomes were best in patients who had higher plasma concentrations of tirilazad at day 4 after treatment. Data on the area under the curve (AUC) in these patients also showed that those on anticonvulsants had significantly less total tirilazad exposure than those not on anticonvulsants (4972 vs. 9704 ng · hr/mL). The AUC for the active tirilazad metabolite was about four times higher for those not on anticonvulsants. Phenytoin is known to induce tirilazad metabolism [20].

Conclusion

Clearly, we have a long way to go in understanding how to best employ cytoprotective therapy, but it is clear that cytoprotection should have a role in the treatment of subarachnoid hemorrhage. Older drugs such as nimodipine and nicardipine exert neuroprotective effects either through effects on calcium activity or by direct neuroprotection. Newer agents such as tirilazad reduce the concentrations of damaging free radicals and can exert a modest preventive action or ameliorate vasospasm after SAH, and this translates into improved outcomes and decreased mortality.

References

1. Hall ED (1995) Inhibition of lipid peroxidation in central nervous system trauma and ischemia. J Neurological Sciences 134 Suppl:79–83
2. Medele RJ, Stummer W, Reulen EIJ, et al (1996) Evidence for peroxidative damage by nitric oxide in experimental chronic cerebral vasospasm. Neurological Research 18(3):277–280
3. Hall ED (1996) Efficacy and mechanism of action of the cytoprotective lipid peroxidation inhibitor tirilazad mesylate in subarachnoid hemorrhage. Eur J Anaesthesiology 13(3): 279–289
4. Gaetani P, Rodriguez y Baena R, Quaglini S, et al (1994) Experimental subarachnoid hemorrhage: events related to antioxidant enzymatic systems and eicosanoid peroxide enhancement. Neurochemical Research 19(7):839–844

5. Macdonald RL, Weir BE (1994) Cerebral vasospasm and free radicals. Free Radical Biology & Medicine 16(5):633–643
6. Gelmers HJ, Hennerici M (1990) Effect of nimodipine on acute ischemic stroke. Pooled results from five randomized trials. Stroke 21:IV81–84
7. Haley EC Jr, Kassell NF, Torner JC, et al (1994) A randomized trial of two doses of nicardipine in aneurysmal subarachnoid hemorrhage. A report of the Cooperative Aneurysm Study. J Neurosurgery 80(5):788–796
8. Hongo R, Kobayashi S (1993) Calcium antagonists for the treatment of vasospasm following subarachnoid hemorrhage. Neurological Research 15(4):218–224
9. Philippon J, Grob R, Dagreou F, Guggiari M, Rivierez M Viars P (1986) Prevention of vasospasm in subarachnoid haemorrhage. A controlled study with nimodipine. Acta Neurochirurgica (Wien) 82(3–4):110–114
10. Barker FG 2nd, Ogilvy CS (1996) Efficacy of prophylactic nimodipine for delayed ischemic deficit after subarachnoid hemorrhage: a metaanalysis. J Neurosurg 84(3):405–414
11. Shibuya M, Suzuki Y, Enomoto H et al (1994) Effects of prophylactic intrathecal administrations of nicardipine on vasospasm in patients with severe aneurysmal subarachnoid hemorrhage. Acta Neurochirurgica (Wien) 131(1–2):19–25
12. Haley EC Jr, Kassell NF, Torner JC, and the participants (1993) A randomized controlled trial of high-dose intravenous nicardipine in aneurysmal subarachnoid hemorrhage. J Neurosurgery 78(4):537–547
13. Young B, Runge JW, Waxman KS, et al (1996) Effects of pegorgotein on neurologic outcome of patients with severe head injury. A multicenter, randomized controlled trial. JAMA 276(7):538–543
14. Gillbe CE, Sage FJ, Gutteridge JM (1996) Commentary. Mannitol: molecule magnifique or a case of radical misinterpretation? Free Radical Research 24(1):1–7
15. Reznick AZ, Kagan VE, Ramsey R, et al (1992) Antiradical effects in L-propionyl carnitine protection of the heart against ischemia-reperfusion injury: the possible role of iron chelation. Arch Biochem Biophys 296(2):394–401
16. Movahed A, Nair KG, Ashavaid TF, Kumar P (1996) Free radical generation and the role of allopurinol as a cardioprotective agent during coronary artery bypass grafting surgery. Can J Cardiol 12(2):138–144
17. Hoffman SW, Moore S, Ellis EF (1997) Isoprostanes: free radical-generated prostaglandins with constrictor effects on cerebral arterioles. Stroke 28(4):844–849
18. Kassell NF, Haley EC Jr, Apperson-Hansen C, et al (1996) Randomized, double-blind, vehicle-controlled trial of tirilazad mesylate in patients with aneurysmal subarachnoid hemorrhage: a cooperative study in Europe, Australia, and New Zealand. J Neurosurgery 84(2):221–228
19. Haley EC Jr, Kassell NF, Apperson-Hansen C, et al (1997) A randomized, double-blind, vehiclecontrolled trial of tirilazad mesylate in patients with aneurysmal subarachnoid hemorrhage: a cooperative study in North America. J Neurosurgery 86(3):467–474
20. Fleishaker JC, Hurst LK, Peters GR (1994) The effect of phenytoin on the pharmacokinetics of tirilazad mesylate in healthy male volunteers. Clinical Pharmacology & Therapeutics S6(4):389–397

Subject Index

MIX
Papier aus verantwortungsvollen Quellen
Paper from responsible sources
FSC® C105338

If you have any concerns about our products,
you can contact us on
ProductSafety@springernature.com

In case Publisher is established outside the EU,
the EU authorized representative is:
Springer Nature Customer Service Center GmbH
Europaplatz 3, 69115 Heidelberg, Germany

Printed by Libri Plureos GmbH
in Hamburg, Germany